OSTEOARTHRITIS
101

A Doctor's Guide for Taking Care of your Knees

OSTEOARTHRITIS
101

A Doctor's Guide for Taking Care of your Knees

Eshwar Kapur, M.D.
with selected illustrations by Mohesh K. Mohan

TABLE OF CONTENTS

DISCLAIMER

My intention is only to provide background information as a means for helping to educate people about general principles of knee osteoarthritis. Everyone, including and especially those who read this book, must seek medical advice, consultation, evaluation, diagnosis, and treatment from a qualified, licensed physician with appropriate training and experience.

This book is not intended to evaluate, diagnose, or treat anyone for any specific medical condition. The written and illustrative contents of this book are for information and education only. Neither the author or publisher, nor any authors, contributors, or other representatives connected to this book will be liable for damages arising out of or in connection with the use of this book. This is a comprehensive limitation of liability that applies to all damages of any kind, including (without limitation) compensatory; direct, indirect or consequential damages; loss of data, income or profit; loss of or damage to property and claims of third parties.

This book should never in any way delay or substitute for seeking medical care for any medical condition. This book does not make any assertion or assumption of your medical diagnoses. The information in this book is for general information purposes and nothing contained in it is, or is intended to be, construed as personal medical advice. It cannot and does not take into account your individual health, medical, physical or emotional situation or needs. This book makes no assessment of any individual's fitness for physical activity, and cannot account for medical allergies or contraindications. It is not a substitute for medical attention, treatment, examination, advice, treatment of existing conditions, or diagnosis, and is not intended to provide a clinical diagnosis nor take the place of proper medical advice from a fully qualified licensed medical practitioner. You should, before you consider any of the information contained in this book, discuss your medical conditions and diagnoses with your doctors. You are responsible for consulting a suitable medical professional before trying any treatment or taking any course of action that may directly or indirectly affect your health or well-being. Any medical care that you pursue is done so solely at your own risk.

The contents of this book should be accurate, based on current research and standard of care related to consensus and generally accepted guidelines, but can become outdated with continuing real-time advancements in medical knowledge. The order of information presented does not in any way indicate prioritization, preference, or endorsement of any diagnostic test or treatment option or protocol. Every individual who reads any parts of this book acknowledges the above disclaimer in full without exception.

SPECIAL DEDICATION

I dedicate this book to my dear mother Sunita Kapur, who poured her heart and soul into raising me and my brother. As the matriarch of our immigrant family integrating into American society during an era of cultural growing pains, my mother was unwavering in ensuring that we would have the best chance possible to achieve our goals and dreams. She is a true humanitarian, with a special interest in writing as a medium for helping people. I am hoping to develop this skill from this first humble effort onwards. I love you Mom— thank you for inspiring me.

Oh, and while we are at it-- I also should thank my father Arun and my brother Anand (also a physician) for assisting me in the editing process. My wife Pearl- thanks for reminding me to stay focused.

And to my dear auntie Yamuna, a general practice physician, thanks for providing the childhood spark that led me to medicine.

INTRODUCTION

I regularly witness the range of negative emotions that patients experience when first diagnosed with osteoarthritis (OA) of the knee. Feelings like anger, disappointment, fear, and worry can become overwhelming. People immediately focus on worst-case scenarios:

"My pain is never going to go away."
"I am going to have to quit my favorite activities forever."
"I am going to end up in a wheelchair."
"I am going to lose my independence."

But knee OA is not necessarily the doomsday diagnosis for physical activities that it once was. There is hope! Whether your OA is mild, moderate, or severe, modern remedies and solutions can help keep you on your feet and preserve your quality of life.

However, I find that too many patients do not know how to get the most from their arthritic knees. The trouble starts because they do not understand knee OA. Education is absolutely necessary for proper care and successful management of your knees. First, you need to know what OA is and what is causing it. This makes you more aware of what you can do to prevent your knees from getting worse. Next, learn everything you can about OA treatment options that can help reduce, eliminate, or reverse your symptoms. There are many medical treatments, but people do not realize their lifestyle habits can have the biggest role in helping or hurting their knees. Finally, once you are an educated and informed patient, you can collaborate with your medical team to take action.

You would figure that your doctors can do all of the above for you: educate you, discuss your treatment options, and devise a comprehensive plan. But the average medical office visit, even with a specialist, is not patient friendly. The time reserved for your doctor's appointment is terribly short, usually just 15 or 30 minutes. That is barely enough time to explain your diagnosis and answer a few of your questions. Making matters worse, in this rushed encounter your doctors may not communicate in plain terms that you can understand. If you don't take notes, you may forget most of what is discussed anyway. It takes a lot of effort to tell you everything you need to know about knee OA, so your doctor typically focuses on a short list of conventional medical treatments like injections, medications, and surgery. Although lifestyle factors like obesity are very influential in knee health, they get unfairly downplayed when they are skipped or barely mentioned.

Many patients leave their doctor's offices feeling overwhelmed with their condition and underwhelmed with the attention they received. Feeling unsupported, they look for other sources of information. They talk to family and friends, go online, and/or search for alternative treatments and "miracle cures". This can lead to the most confusion and misinformation.

I wrote this book so that basic, reliable, comprehensive information about knee OA that you need is available beyond what you will get in a trip to your doctor's office. I have gathered frequently asked questions from the thousands of patients I have seen. The answers are simple and straightforward, based on science. The goal is to offer the education you need:

- You will learn about arthritis.
- You will learn about how to navigate your doctor's visits to ensure an accurate diagnosis.
- You will learn about immediate and long-term strategies to reduce knee pain and improve function.

In this book, you will notice an effort to emphasize the fact that your daily habits are just as important as medical treatments. The way you care for your knees (and your body) from morning to evening is critical.

Once you read this book, you will be better informed. Rather than relying on your doctor to make decisions, you will be empowered as an educated healthcare consumer. You should be able to have better, higher quality discussions with your medical team. You will be able to partner with your medical providers to create a plan of action on your terms.

And remember, although this book is designed to educate you, it is not intended to diagnose or treat a medical condition. Therefore, this book does not in any way replace the need for you to see your doctor for evaluation and treatment for general knee pain, osteoarthritis, or whatever else ails you. All treatments mentioned in this book must be approved by a medical professional directly involved in your healthcare. Thank you!

CHAPTER 1
WHAT IS OSTEOARTHRITIS?

I want to know what treatments I can try for my osteoarthritis. Where do we begin?

Knowledge is the first step in empowering yourself to get what you want: reduce pain and stay active. Let's start by understanding what is happening "behind the scenes" in your knees so that your treatment decisions will make better sense to you. Knowledge will make you a more educated patient, and you will be a more active participant in your care. You will have better control of your health and well-being.

What can cause my knee to hurt?

The knee joint is made from bones, muscles, ligaments, and cartilage. Let's explore the basic structure of the knee.

Bones come together to form the structure of the joint. There are 4 bones: the *patella* (kneecap), *femur* (thighbone), *tibia* (big shinbone), and *fibula* (small shinbone).

Ligaments are thick bands of tissue that connect the bones together to keep the joint from falling apart.

Muscles move bones in different directions. Thickened muscle ends called tendons connect the muscles to the bones. For the knee, there are 2 main movements- flexion (bend the knee) and extension (extend the knee).

Cartilage sits between the bones in the knee to absorb shock, stabilize the joint, and allow for smooth movement.

Any of these structures could become painful. For example:

Bones can become fractured (broken) or bruised with a sudden trauma or with gradual overuse. The injured bone becomes very tender and there is often difficulty in weightbearing.

Ligaments get torn or stretched with an awkward twist or collision. A ligament injury is obvious and easy to diagnose.

Muscles and tendons can tear partially or completely, suddenly or gradually with time. These injuries are easy to diagnose because the pain is either obviously in the muscle or exactly where a tendon attaches to bone.

Cartilage can tear suddenly or get damaged over time. There will be pain in the joint on either side of the knee or under the kneecap. When someone says "my knee is worn out", it usually means that their cartilage is damaged. *Cartilage breakdown is the main cause of osteoarthritis.*

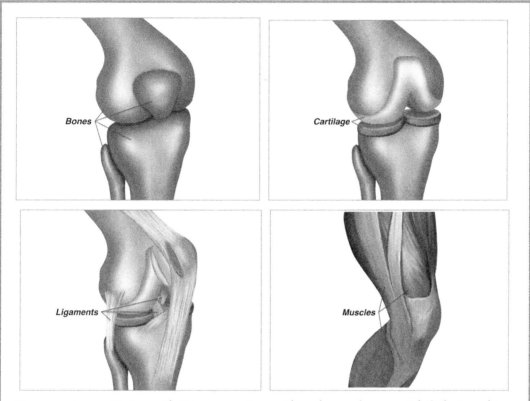

Knee anatomy. Osteoarthritis occurs in cartilage layers (upper right) that cushion and protect the joint. The bones form the joint, the ligaments hold the bones together, and the muscles move the joint.

What is arthritis?

Arthritis is a medical term that means "inflammation in the joint".

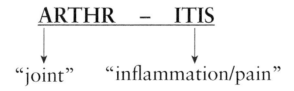

ARTHR – ITIS

"joint"   "inflammation/pain"

Inflammation is a tool that our immune systems use to try to heal the body when confronted with injuries, infections, or other "threats". Inflammation brings in fluid, chemicals, and repair cells to the affected area. Strong pain signals are created as part of the inflammatory process, to make us fully aware that there is a problem.

Arthritis is a specific term to indicate inflammation in any joint in the body. However, there are hundreds of specific types of arthritis, depending on what causes the inflammation.

What are some examples of arthritis?

There are many types of arthritis. Each has a different cause, depending on what provokes the inflammation in a joint space. Arthritis may affect one or many joints. Here are some common examples:

Septic arthritis: Infection causes a very dangerous condition called "septic arthritis", which will usually affect one joint. The infection is caused by a microorganism such as a virus or bacteria that gets into a joint. This can happen from direct entrance from the outside when a trauma occurs. Other causes include ongoing infection elsewhere in the body that spreads into the joint. Symptoms of septic arthritis are sudden onset of swelling, redness, and extreme pain with even small movements, often accompanied by fever and malaise. Septic arthritis requires aggressive treatment with antibiotics. Often, surgery is needed to clean out the infected joint. This is a very dangerous form of arthritis because catastrophic outcomes including death can occur within days if not properly treated.

Rheumatoid arthritis: Rheumatoid arthritis(RA) is a painful, destructive condition where a person's immune system attacks his/her own joints. RA is often diagnosed and treated by rheumatologists, often with the help of blood tests and x-rays. Typically, RA affects many joints at once on both sides of the body, especially the hands. Over time, RA's persistent assault on the joints can lead to devastating, debilitating joint deformities. Fortunately, there are treatments that can control and sometimes stop RA from destroying the joints.

Gouty arthritis (gout): Gout is an arthritic condition related to food consumption. Purines found in alcohol, certain meats, and seafood break down during digestion and form a waste product called uric acid. Some people cannot get rid of uric acid fast enough, causing it to accumulate in the blood. When it reaches a high level, the uric acid turns into crystals that deposit into joints, causing sudden, severe pain and swelling. This is known as a "gout attack", which will usually involve one joint per episode. Gout causes extremely painful inflammation that is treated with anti-inflammatory medications, but can last for days or weeks. Gout attacks can be prevented with strict diet modifications, with or without the help of medications. Recurring gout episodes can lead to joint destruction and chronic pain.

Osteoarthritis is *the most common type of arthritis*, and is also the most common cause of chronic knee pain. It is a term for the pain that occurs when a joint has "wear and tear" from degenerative joint disease. This is the arthritis that is associated with "getting older in age".

In this book, we will be focusing on osteoarthritis!

What is degenerative joint disease, and how is it related to osteoarthritis?

Basically, degenerative joint disease means that there is "wear and tear" in a joint. Degenerative joint disease is NOT always painful. When the "wear and tear" of degenerative joint disease causes pain, it is called osteoarthritis.

Exactly where in the knee does "wear and tear" occur that causes osteoarthritis pain?

"Wear and tear" in degenerative joint disease occurs in the cartilage that sits between the bones in the joint. As degenerative disease worsens, the bones themselves get damaged.

What is cartilage and what is its purpose?

Cartilage is thick, soft, smooth body tissue. There are two types of cartilage in the knee joint. There is thin *articular cartilage* that lines the bones of virtually all joints. Unique to the knee, there is also *meniscus cartilage* that sits between the bones. These protective cartilage layers work together to absorb shock and make movement smooth and frictionless. The meniscus tissue also adds stability to knee joints.

What exactly happens to the cartilage in degenerative joint disease?

In degenerative joint disease, the cartilage protecting the knee joint becomes permanently damaged. This may start early in life with accidents or sports injuries that cause tears that do not heal perfectly. Meanwhile, as we get older, cartilage naturally weakens and gets worn out more easily. Overall, tears, frayed ends, fissures, rough surfaces, and tissue loss accumulate. The joint loses its ability to absorb shock and move smoothly. As time goes on, the cartilage continues to disintegrate and rub away. With the loss of the protective cartilage layers, the knee joint starts to collapse until it becomes "bone to bone".

Does "wear and tear" always cause pain?

Thankfully, no-- you can have "wear and tear" without pain. The cartilage does not have to be in perfect condition for the knee to function. However, with damaged cartilage, the joint becomes less durable. The knees have less protection and get irritated more easily with less activity. As the "wear and tear" gets worse over time and the bones start to rub together, it becomes more likely that pain will occur.

How does degenerative joint disease turn into osteoarthritis?

With damaged, worn out cartilage, the degenerative joint has less cushioning protection. Stress builds up more easily with less activity. When joint stress reaches a critical level, complex chemical pathways get triggered that lead to painful inflammation. This process leading to pain defines osteoarthritis. Osteoarthritis is the painful condition that occurs when a degenerative joint becomes aggravated.

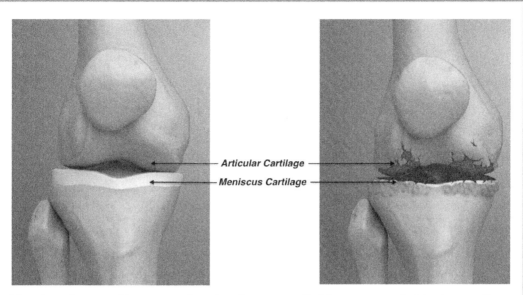

Here is an image of intact cartilage in a knee joint (left). In osteoarthritis, the cartilage is severely damaged, with tearing, frayed ends, fissures, and lost tissue (right).

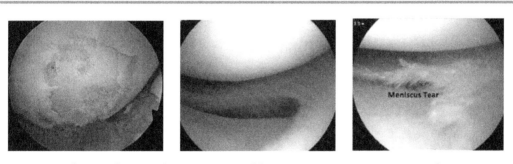

Damaged articular cartilage   Normal knee joint   Meniscus cartilage tears

Interior of the knee joint, seen during surgery

Arthroscopic look (camera view) of the inside of the knee joint, showing cartilage damage.

My doctors keep saying I have osteoarthritis- but is it possible I have a torn meniscus?

Yes! Osteoarthritis is caused by damaged cartilage in the joint, which often includes severe tearing in the meniscus. We will discuss this later.

Why does cartilage damage occur?

Cartilage in the knee constantly absorbs stress in small amounts each day through routine use in sports, repetitive work, and general overuse. Meanwhile, accidents and injuries causing the knee to become abnormally bent or twisted can cause sudden, permanent cartilage loss. When we are young, our bodies can repair cartilage to a certain extent. However, as we get older, cartilage heals less, and damage accumulates.

There are several factors that can determine how long our bodies can maintain healthy cartilage. Obesity, chronic medical problems, poor diet, genetics, and bad lifestyle habits can all accelerate or contribute to degenerative joint disease.

Is there a cure for osteoarthritis(OA)?

No— OA is a condition that is irreversible. This is because the cartilage damage in degenerative joint disease becomes complex and extensive, typically beyond repair. As cartilage wears out, there is a loss of space between the bones that can never be recovered. This can progress to "bone on bone" joint collapse, the hallmark of severe OA.

CHAPTER 2
MAKING THE DIAGNOSIS

Osteoarthritis is the most common cause of chronic knee pain, especially for people over 50 years old. If you have knee pain and your x-rays show evidence of "wear and tear", then it is extremely likely that you have osteoarthritis. But knee pain has other causes to consider, especially if you have normal x-rays and/or if there was a recent injury. Your goal is to get the definitive answer to the question: "what is my diagnosis?" Simple cases may only require one office visit with your family doctor to confirm your diagnosis. However, in many scenarios, you may need to see a "bone and joint" specialist or have a series of tests done to get the answer. In this section, you will learn how you and your doctors can team up to figure out what is causing your knee pain.

How does your doctor properly diagnose osteoarthritis(OA)?

There is no single test that will diagnose OA. The diagnosis can be confirmed with information from 3 main sources:

1. **Your history**- You will be asked a series of specific questions about your knee pain to see if you have typical OA symptoms. Your doctor will also inquire about your general medical history to check for other causes of knee pain.

2. **Your physical examination**- Your doctor will examine your knee for tenderness, instability, swelling, and stiffness.

3. **Your diagnostic imaging**- x-rays are excellent at detecting the presence of degenerative joint disease that causes osteoarthritis pain. If your x-rays are normal, you may need other imaging tests.

During your evaluation, the information above will be used by your doctor to also consider all causes of knee pain. Your doctor will seek answers to the following:

- Is a muscle or tendon that moves the joint torn or injured?
- Is a ligament that keeps the bones connected to each other torn or injured?
- Is a bone broken, injured, or otherwise abnormal?
- If there is arthritis in the joint, what kind is it?
- Is there something weird/uncommon going on?

How does my history help predict the cause of my knee pain?

The story that you tell about your knee pain can be very helpful for your doctor in figuring out what is wrong. If you are vague and disorganized, the process is much harder. The more details you communicate, the better. Get ready to summarize your general medical history. With your knee pain, think about how long you have been having symptoms. Create a timeline that starts when you first developed knee pain and how it has changed.

Your doctor will also want other details about your knee pain:
- when and where the knee hurts
- what kind of pain you have
- what movements are painful
- what your activity limitations are
- feelings of instability
- etc.

Your doctor will use the information you provide to help solve the mystery. For example, a history of a trauma that has led to instability would make your doctor concerned about a ligament injury. A sudden injury during exercise leading to immediate weakness would raise suspicion for a torn muscle. An injury that came on gradually with a new or consistent activity could be from several causes.

A great office visit requires an organized patient paired with an attentive doctor who is appropriately engaged. On your end, bring your best. Write notes ahead of time and bring them with you when you see your doctor. This sample questionnaire can help get you organized.

KNEE PAIN QUESTIONNAIRE

How long have you had this pain/condition? _____

Was there an injury or trauma? ☐NO ☐YES—please describe: _____
_____

HAVE YOU HAD SURGERY IN THIS KNEE? ☐NO ☐YES, year(s)_____

Location of pain:	Describe the pain:	Does the pain radiate:	Is the pain:
☐front ☐back ☐side ☐other _____	☐sharp pain ☐dull ache ☐burning ☐numbness ☐tingling ☐other____	☐NO ☐YES, to_____	☐ mild/annoying ☐ medium/distracting ☐ severe/disabling

Do you have any associated symptoms?	When do you get the pain?		
☐weakness ☐clicking ☐locking ☐stiffness ☐feeling of instability ☐other_____	☐walking ☐twist/turning ☐bend/squatting	☐running ☐sitting ☐"all the time"	☐standing ☐stairs/hills

Have you RECENTLY had a "cortisone" injection for this problem? ☐NO ☐YES, date_____ -- Have you EVER had a "cortisone" injection in this joint/area? ☐NO ☐YES	OCCUPATION: _____ ☐I'm retired! Do you use tobacco? ☐NO ☐YES

TREATMENT YOU HAVE TRIED SO FAR:

Physical therapy	☐NO ☐YES, how many sessions?_____	
Medications	☐NO ☐YES, which medications?_____	
Ice	☐NO ☐YES	Heat ☐NO ☐YES
Other treatments	_____ _____ _____	

OTHER SYMPTOMS: *If you check any of the items here, please schedule an appointment with your primary care physician to review.*

☐Chest pain	☐Nausea	☐Difficulty breathing	☐Cough	☐Shortness of breath
☐Night sweats	☐Vomiting	☐Abdominal pain	☐Fever	☐Weight loss

Please list your TYPICAL weekly activities:

ACTIVITY	MINUTES/ SESSION	DAYS PER WEEK (CIRCLE)	DID YOU STOP THIS ACTIVITY BECAUSE OF YOUR INJURY?
		S S M T W R F	☐YES ☐NO
		S S M T W R F	☐YES ☐NO
		S S M T W R F	☐YES ☐NO
		S S M T W R F	☐YES ☐NO

This worksheet can help get your knee pain symptoms and history together in detail.

What are typical symptoms of osteoarthritis (OA)?

OA is the most common cause of **chronic knee pain.** There are typical pain features, with some variability. Often, the pain is located along one or both sides of the knee. Patients may also indicate that the pain is in front of the knee, under the kneecap, or "all over". The pain is usually dull and achy, but when severe it may become sharp at times. The pain tends to build up gradually over weeks, months, or years and may constantly wax and wane. However, traumas or quick increases in activity may cause sudden OA flare-ups. The pain is usually worse with weightbearing physical activities. But patients may report discomfort when stationary with prolonged sitting or lying down (sleeping). Other common features of OA knee pain:

- Age is typically over 40 years old.
- There can be cracking, popping, pinching,or "catching" sensations in the joint.
- There may be a loss of range of motion in the knee, with inability to fully bend, extend, or both.
- Pain can occur in one or both knees, and one may be worse than the other.
- Joint swelling ("water on the knee") can occur. This often causes a sensation of stiffness.

What symptoms are NOT typical for osteoarthritis(OA)?

If you have the following symptoms, other conditions besides OA are likely and must be considered. You may need a series of tests, or a visit with a specialist to sort out your diagnosis, even if you have x-rays suggestive of degenerative joint disease:

- **Sudden severe pain:** If there was a trauma, accident, twist, or fall, an injury should be considered. There could be a broken bone, torn muscle, or sprained ligament. Sudden pain without an injury should lead your doctor to consider an inflammatory medical condition like gout or joint infection.

- **Instability:** A "loose" knee that seems to collapse or buckle with certain movements may indicate torn ligaments, excessive kneecap laxity, or severe meniscus tears.

- **Radiating pain:** Knee problems do not typically cause pain that radiates up the thigh or down the shin to the foot/ankle. In this case, your doctor should examine your spine and entire leg, and you may need nerve testing as well.

- **Numbness/tingling:** Knee OA does not cause numbness and/or tingling. If you have such symptoms, especially if there is also leg weakness, your knee pain may be a symptom of a nerve problem.

- **Swelling in both knees:** It is true that knee OA may cause joint swelling, and at any given time the swelling may be in one or both knees. However, consistent obvious swelling or "water" in both knees may indicate a problem other than OA. Your doctor may discuss further testing that could include fluid analysis and bloodwork.

- **Pain in other joints:** Widespread pain in several joints in the body, or the feeling that you are sore "all over", could indicate other types of arthritis besides OA. Pain in many joints in a symmetric pattern involving both sides of the body may be particularly concerning.

- **General symptoms:** Fever, weight loss, and fatigue are not directly associated with OA. If you have joint pain but are also generally feeling unwell, make sure you let your doctor know.

How does my physical examination reveal osteoarthritis(OA)?

A physical examination of your knee is necessary to confirm your diagnosis. Patients are sometimes diagnosed with osteoarthritis based on age or x-ray findings. However, your doctor should not and cannot say you have osteoarthritis without examining you.

There are several physical findings to help diagnose OA. Your doctor will do the following to collect information that will help determine what is causing your knee pain:

Palpation- your doctor will systematically feel the various muscles, tendons, ligaments, and bones in and around the knee. This is called *palpation*, useful for detecting tenderness, swelling, abnormal lumps/bumps, etc. OA specifically causes tenderness on the sides of the joint or around the kneecap. Your doctor may also find swelling in an arthritic joint, as inflammation can cause a fluid buildup.

Movement- it is important for your doctor to bend and straighten the knee to check for how well the joint is able to move. Many conditions, including knee OA, will cause limitations in movement either from pain, stiffness, or both.

Strength- Your doctor may ask you to bend or extend your knees against resistance to test the strength of the muscles that support the joint.

Provocative measures- Your doctor should put your knees through a quick series of special tests where your knee will be gently twisted, wiggled, and moved in various ways. Each test gives your doctor specific information to assist with your diagnosis.

What tests do I need to diagnose knee osteoarthritis(OA)?

1. **Diagnostic imaging**: Imaging studies produce pictures to visualize the internal structures of the knees. X-rays can clearly identify the degenerative changes that cause OA. **Therefore, an x-ray should be done in all evaluations for osteoarthritis.** In some cases, especially if your x-rays are normal, other imaging tests such as MRI, CT scanning, or ultrasound may be needed.

2. **Blood testing:** Knee pain is most often related to structural damage in or around the joints. In these cases, when something is sprained, strained, torn, broken, or wearing out, blood testing is not usually needed. However, if the knee is structurally intact, then your doctor may look into your medical history more closely. If a medical disease is suspected as a cause of your knee pain, you may be given the option to get bloodwork. Blood

testing can identify conditions such as gout, infection, rheumatoid arthritis, lupus, etc.

3. **Fluid analysis:** If the knee joint is swollen, examination of the fluid can provide important information for your diagnosis. This requires a simple procedure done at your doctor's office. A fluid sample is extracted from the joint with a small needle, and sent to the lab for analysis. Although OA doesn't have any telltale fluid findings, gout and other types of arthritis do have characteristic fluid components. Fluid analysis has to be done if infection is suspected. In the case of a major trauma or injury, swelling is expected and fluid extraction may not be needed.

How do doctors "see" osteoarthritis(OA) if the damage is internal?

As cartilage wears out in degenerative joint disease that leads to OA, the space between the bones in the knee joint becomes narrow. The worse the cartilage is damaged, the smaller the space gets, until the cartilage is completely destroyed and the joint collapses, becoming "bone on bone". Even though cartilage is not actually visible, x-ray is the best imaging test for measuring the loss of joint space. When x-rays are normal, this means that that the joint space is preserved, but cartilage may still be damaged. If degenerative joint disease is still suspected, then MRI can be done to "see" the cartilage damage more directly. MRI, therefore, can detect degenerative joint disease when the x-rays look normal. It is important to know that MRI cannot measure joint space loss. Therefore, even if an MRI is done first, x-rays are needed to get a complete assessment of your knees.

Do x-rays really show anything?

Yes! X-rays are generally very useful in the evaluation of knee pain and show much more than patients realize. People seem to think that x-rays are only good for showing broken bones. However, x-rays give doctors plenty of information. Bone disease, ligament tears, and cartilage damage can be seen on x-rays. X-ray is the only imaging test that can determine joint space loss that defines degenerative joint disease that causes osteoarthritis. Therefore, x-rays are always needed when osteoarthritis is suspected.

What does osteoarthritis look like on x-ray?

X-rays show several findings that can confirm the presence of degenerative joint disease that leads to osteoarthritis. It is important that the x-rays are done properly.

1. **WEIGHTBEARING FRONTAL VIEW X-RAYS** are taken with you standing in front of the x-ray machine. You see the bones of the knee as if you are looking in the mirror. This x-ray view shows the loss of joint space that occurs when cartilage gets damaged in osteoarthritis. As degenerative joint disease worsens, the bones get closer together until the knee becomes "bone on bone".

   Other findings to suggest osteoarthritis include bone spurs (osteophytes) from poor healing, as well as cysts under the bone surface of the joint where fluid has seeped in because of a lack of cartilage.

   Frontal views can be done with you standing straight or standing with your knees slightly bent. Your doctor may suggest either view or both to be done.

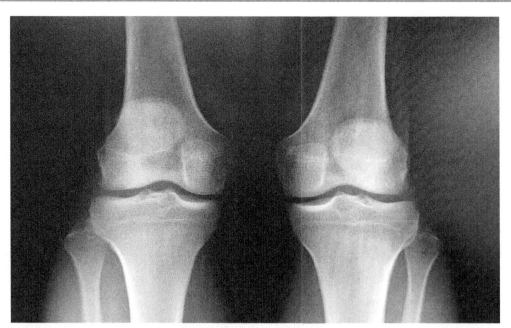

Frontal view x-ray. The knees are oriented as though the patient is standing in front of you. This is the most informative x-ray view for knee osteoarthritis.

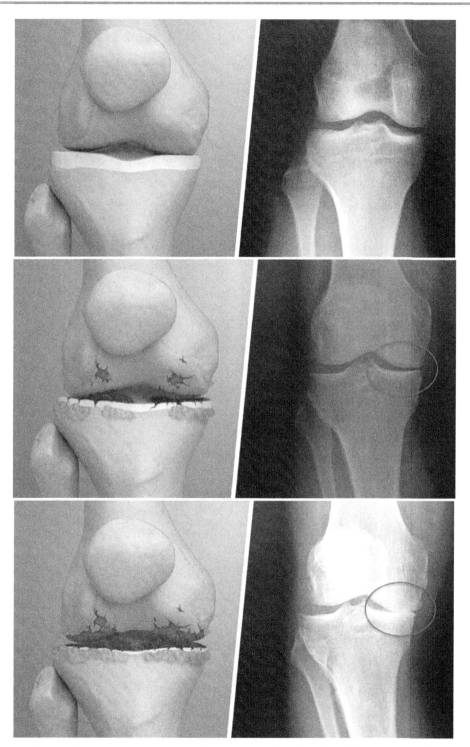

As cartilage damage gets worse in osteoarthritis, the joint space decreases (*red ovals*). This is seen most clearly on frontal weightbearing x-rays.

2. **LATERAL views** show the knee joint from the side. Here, loss of joint space can be assessed in the patellofemoral (kneecap) joint.

3. **SPECIAL KNEECAP** (Merchant) views are very important and often overlooked. Merchant views are the best x-rays to check the patellofemoral (kneecap) joint space for degenerative joint disease. Bone spurs are often seen here as well. These views are also generally excellent in showing how well the kneecap sits on the thighbone. Kneecap alignment can contribute to chronic knee pain and instability over a lifetime.

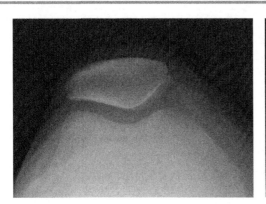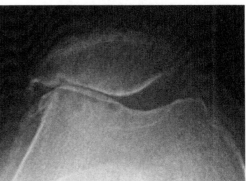

Merchant view x-rays show the patellofemoral (kneecap) joint, where osteoarthritis can occur when cartilage between the bones is damaged and joint space is lost (right).

By examining your x-rays, your doctor can estimate the extent of degenerative joint disease by measuring the amount of joint space loss:

+ Mild (less than 50 percent loss of joint space)

++ Moderate (50-90 percent loss of joint space)

+++ Severe (90+ percent loss of joint space/"bone-on-bone")

If your doctor just says "your x-rays show that you have arthritis", ask "how bad is the 'wear and tear'? Mild, moderate, or severe?"

My X-rays were NOT weightbearing- is that OK?

No, it is not OK. When you are standing, your weight compresses the joint and shows reduced space most accurately. Loss of space between the bones in the joint is the key x-ray finding that helps to confirm if you have osteoarthritis. If you are not weightbearing (standing) for the frontal x-ray, arthritic joints may look normal.

I did not have the special kneecap view—is that OK?

NO! A small percentage of people only have OA in the kneecap joints. Therefore, the kneecap (Merchants) views must be included in all workups for chronic knee pain to check for loss of joint space in this often-missed area.

Do I need an MRI to diagnose osteoarthritis?

Probably not...but maybe! When there is joint space loss on the x-ray, we already know the cartilage is extensively damaged, and your chronic knee pain is very likely coming from degenerative joint disease (DJD)/osteoarthritis. Once an x-ray shows moderate or severe DJD, your knee is usually past the point of MRI, so further imaging is rarely needed. Occasionally, your doctor may be concerned about a different diagnosis even if your x-rays suggest osteoarthritis. In this rare scenario, you may need further testing like an MRI.

If your x-rays look normal, then your diagnosis may be unclear and an MRI can be useful. MRI can detect early "wear and tear" in the knee joint before it shows up on an x-ray. MRI can also help confirm or rule out other diagnoses. Keep in mind that MRI is not always the best test after x-ray. Ultrasound, CT scan, or bone scan may be better, depending on what your doctor thinks is going on. You may even need several tests to completely figure things out.

Which specialist should I ask for?

Osteoarthritis (OA) can be diagnosed and treated by your regular primary care physician. However, there can be a few challenges to consider. If your doctor is helping you with a lot of other medical problems, there may not be enough time to properly focus on your joints. Also, musculoskeletal medicine is an admitted weakness for many primary care physicians, and they may not feel comfortable counseling you about your knee pain. Also consider that your family doctor may be able to offer some treatment, but may not be aware of all your options. The primary care physician is a good first resource, at least to get your evaluation started. In many insurance plans, you are required to see your primary care provider before seeing a specialist. At any point, if you feel like you need more treatment or information than what your doctor is offering, ask to see a specialist.

Which specialist should you choose? There are several options. Each type of specialist has a slightly different approach and expertise. With an empowerment strategy, you are the coordinator of your care. You can entrust one specialist for your care, or build a team as you wish. Start with one physician and see how it goes. You may need a second opinion within the same specialty, or you may seek advice from several different types of specialists. You may reserve a spot on your medical team for a particular doctor for a specific treatment. For complex situations or whenever your diagnosis is unclear, you may need input from several physicians.

Your options for specialists include orthopedic surgeons, sports medicine physicians, and rheumatologists.

Orthopedic surgeons diagnose and treat structural problems with muscles, bones, and joints. They are generally considered experts in the care of osteoarthritis, but may tend to focus on surgical options.

There are 3 types of knee orthopedists:
- *Joint surgeons* specialize in performing knee replacement surgery for patients with severe OA that have failed nonsurgical treatments.

- *Sports medicine surgeons* focus on athletic injuries, but will tend to see some OA patients. Active people with OA who may be too young for a knee replacement can see a sports surgeon to find out if there are other surgical options.

- *General orthopedic surgeons* do not have specialty certification for sports or joint surgery. If your community does not have specialized joint or sports surgeons, then you may end up seeing a generalist. Their skillset for arthroscopy and knee replacement surgery may vary tremendously.

Sports medicine physicians have a primary care background and do not perform surgery. They take care of athletes and active individuals for various medical issues, including OA. Primary care sports physicians may be part of a group of family physicians, or may work in an orthopedic group alongside a team of surgeons. These physicians are a good option if you are not a surgical candidate or simply not interested in surgery.

Rheumatologists specialize in various joint disorders, including knee pain, caused by medical problems from within your body. If there is uncertainty about your knee pain, especially if OA does not seem to be the likely cause, then these specialists will provide helpful input. Some rheumatologists may also provide nonsurgical treatment for OA.

Specialists for Osteoarthritis/Knee Pain

Orthopedic Surgeon
- Joint Specialist
- Sports Specialist
- General Orthopedist

Primary Care Sports Medicine Physician
Rheumatologist

CHAPTER 3
COPING WITH OSTEOARTHRITIS

How do I deal with a new diagnosis of osteoarthritis(OA)?

To properly cope with having OA, the first step is to remain positive. It is important to understand that the body is not designed to last forever. Our joints may naturally break down over time, but the process is manageable. There are many treatments and interventions that you can try, to keep you active with less pain. Thinking positive will help maintain proper focus on successful control of your arthritis.

Next, be proactive. Educate yourself with this book and other resources, along with your specialist consultations. Learn everything you can about OA and your treatment options. Develop a strategy for the battle. You have full control in developing an OA action plan. It's really all up to you putting forth your best effort. Some interventions require the help of your medical team, but there are many treatment options that you can try on your own at home. Empower yourself to create a customized pathway for the care of your knees.

Am I really going to be OK?

YES. Osteoarthritis is not a life-threatening condition. There are many ways to improve function and decrease pain. Combined with a smart approach to daily living, most people can find a plan of action that will allow a great quality of life. Every step of the way, there are always options. When you have pain episodes, you may need to simply lay low for a while and try home remedies, or you can see your doctor for medical treatments. Once your knee pain resolves, there are several strategies to help you stay pain-free. And if all else fails, and your osteoarthritis is severe, you can inquire about knee replacement surgery that can "fix" your knee as a last resort.

What are some tips to help me cope with having osteoarthritis (OA)?

- **Learn as much as you can:** take the mystery away from your knee pain by learning all about it. The more familiar you are with OA, the easier it is to manage.

- **Focus on your abilities instead of disabilities:** There is a tendency to get sad about what your OA is keeping you from doing. If you have this "glass is half empty" way of thinking, then try to reverse your focus. Rather than dwelling on your limitations, try to get joy in everything that you are able to do. For instance, instead of being bummed out that you couldn't play 18 holes of golf, learn to be satisfied about getting through 9 holes pain-free. Get it? Stop worrying about what you can't do, and enjoy what you can do on any given day. This is a very powerful way of thinking that will help you conquer your OA.

- **Find new challenges that do not cause knee pain**: Modify your current activities, or find new sports/hobbies that are low impact and low risk.

- **Diversify your interests:** When you have OA, you may find yourself with occasional downtime when your knees are not cooperative. Even if you consider yourself to be an athlete, you should never be overly dependent on physical activities for your happiness. In case you are forced to scale back your athletic pursuits for a while, have at least one "knee-proof" hobby or interest to keep you engaged, entertained and stimulated.

- **Develop a support system of family, friends, and health professionals:** People tend to get isolated by their medical problems when chronic health issues like knee pain cause them to avoid being around others. You may feel like you would rather be alone when your physically not your best, but you can end up depressed and lonely as a result. Try to keep yourself in touch with your social life through simple meetups, phone calls, "family nights", etc. This can prove to be very uplifting and therapeutic. Meanwhile, keep health professionals on standby for whenever you need help managing difficult symptoms.

Quick Tips for Dealing with Osteoarthritis

Be +positive+.

Empower yourself with education!

Focus on your abilities rather than your disability.

Develop a "Support Network".

Diversify your activities and interests.

I feel doomed that I found out that I have osteoarthritis—will I have to quit my favorite activities?

In the past, a diagnosis of osteoarthritis would be a "death sentence" for activity. There was this automatic assumption that a person couldn't possibly exercise with worn out knee joints. But these days, we know that most arthritic knees, especially in mild stages, can still handle physical activity. With reasonable modifications, you should be encouraged to remain involved in most of your favorite sports/hobbies as long as possible.

Can't I just have knee replacement surgery and get it over with now?

This is a great question, and we will talk about the surgery in more detail later. Knee replacement surgery seems like the ultimate cure to get people with OA back to the activities they enjoy. In fact, some people think that a nonsurgical approach is a waste of time if knee replacement surgery will get rid of their pain. It is true, knee replacement is a great option, when the time is right. However, the reality is that the surgery has risks and imperfections, and cannot be undone. Knee replacement surgery performed too early can have unpredictable results and lead to new activity restrictions, triggering dissatisfaction and regrets. Also, the new implant will not last forever, so surgery done early in life may require repeat knee replacement down the line. Every once in a while, the surgical procedure will cause complications that can be serious. Therefore, knee replacement surgery is usually reserved for the final step for severe OA when all else has failed. In the meantime, it is important to give the conservative approach an earnest effort to find a satisfactory "new normal".

There is an appropriate time and place for knee replacement surgery, typically when the knee is completely worn out. Each person's case is unique. See your doctors and they will counsel you about when you should consider surgery based on your situation.

CHAPTER 4
YOUR TREATMENT OPTIONS

What are my treatment options to fight osteoarthritis?

There are several different categories of treatments available for osteoarthritis. Treatment goals include pain control, maintenance of function, and joint preservation. There is no way to reverse joint damage, but it is theoretically possible to slow it down. Although we tend to focus on the medical treatments provided by doctors and surgeons, there is a lot that you can do on your own to successfully control osteoarthritis.

We are going to review your options as follows:

1. **Lifestyle interventions** have been shown to improve osteoarthritis outcomes.
2. **Medical treatments** have a range of benefits for improvements in pain and function.
3. **Surgery** is an option in certain situations.

What are lifestyle changes?

Osteoarthritis is caused by physical activities, accidents, injuries, and traumas that cause sudden or chronic damage to your knees over your lifetime. Meanwhile, there are several lifestyle habits that increase your risk for knee osteoarthritis. By making changes in aspects of your daily life such as occupation, sports/hobbies, nutrition, etc., you could dramatically reduce pain episodes and improve function both day-to-day and in the long term.

What medical treatments are available?

Traditional medical treatments include your doctor's recommendations for self-care. Examples include applying ice and heat, doing physical therapy home exercises, and using over the counter pain medications. Your doctor can also prescribe medications and administer injections. There are several "alternative" medical options that can be prescribed or recommended by your doctor.

What surgical treatments are available for knee osteoarthritis(OA)?

Most people have heard of knee replacement surgery for osteoarthritis. This surgery is the classic procedure for osteoarthritis when all other options have failed. Although knee replacement has some variations, the basic mechanics of the prosthesis and the surgery are very similar.

Osteoarthritis does have other surgical options for certain types of individual situations that depend on age, severity of arthritis, age, symptoms, leg alignment, etc. If you have failed conservative options and your OA knee pain has rendered you nonfunctional, then a consultation with an orthopedic surgeon will be helpful to explore your surgical options. We will discuss surgery for OA in detail later.

Treatment Options for Knee Osteoarthritis

Lifestyle Changes
- **Decrease Risk Factors**
  - Lose weight if overweight/obese
  - Stop smoking
  - Modify Physical Activities
- **Improve Health**
- Eat healthier
- Get better rest (sleep)

Medical Treatments
- Medications/Injections
- Physical therapy
- Alternative treatments

Surgical Treatments
- Knee Replacement Surgery
- Arthroscopic Surgery

CHAPTER 5
LIFESTYLE INTERVENTIONS

How does lifestyle affect my osteoarthritis(OA)?

The way you treat your body from day to day has a huge effect on how your OA will behave. Healthy lifestyle habits can protect your knees, prevent degenerative disease, and maximize your musculoskeletal health. Simple changes in your health can help you control OA pain with less medications, and may be able to slow the disease process down over the years.

Could my lifestyle cause or worsen my knee pain?

Yes. Poor lifestyle habits can accelerate the "wear and tear" process and make osteoarthritis worse both in the short and long term. Some lifestyle factors like sports and labor-based occupations cause excessive physical stress that break down the joints.

Meanwhile, diet, smoking, obesity, and sleep problems can stimulate chronic inflammation. Normally, inflammation is the body's natural defense against infection, illness, and injury. But when inflammation is constantly triggered, it causes painful, destructive damage throughout the body. In OA, chronic inflammation can increase joint aggravation and speed up the "wear and tear" process. Lifestyle changes to improve health and reduce inflammation can save your joints.

Lifestyle interventions are simple and straightforward investments in your health. They are empowering because they put you in control of your outcome. Motivation and effort may be required to undo bad tendencies that may have developed over many years. It is never too late to make changes. Read about the following ways you can manage osteoarthritis risks.

LIFESTYLE INTERVENTION 1: STOP SMOKING (NOW!)

Why is smoking bad for joints?

Cigarette smoke releases numerous chemicals into the body that increases inflammation. This leads to internal chaos that is terrible for health. Smoking is an irritant that can cause or worsen heart disease, cancer, and many other medical conditions, including osteoarthritis. Chronic inflammation from smoking constantly aggravates your joints, while speeding up degenerative disease. In fact, studies have shown that smokers suffer more cartilage loss and have more knee pain than nonsmokers.

Simple Tips to Quit Smoking

- Keep cutting back your total daily use by one cigarette.

- Delay the first cigarette of the day for as long as possible.

- At a time when you would typically smoke, eat a healthy snack instead and then see if you still feel like smoking.

- Look for healthier ways to relieve stress if you normally smoke when you are under pressure.

- Get support with talk therapy, weekly coaching, or online programs designed to help you quit smoking.

If you smoke, put tobacco cessation at the top of your OA treatment plan, for your knees but also for sake of your general health. If you cannot quit right away, start by cutting back to get yourself headed in the right direction. But remember that exposure to as little as one cigarette per day is enough to cause irreversible bodily damage. Talk to your primary care physician, insurance provider, or local hospital system to find out what resources are available to help you quit smoking.

LIFESTYLE INTERVENTION 2: MAINTAIN HEALTHY WEIGHT

Why is obesity dangerous for osteoarthritis?

Obesity means your body mass index (BMI), a calculation that compares your height and weight, is above 30. You can use the chart on the next page to check your BMI. Obesity makes the body dysfunctional and increases risks for many diseases and medical conditions, such as osteoarthritis.

Most people can understand that obesity literally overloads the knees. The physical stress on your knees is quite dramatic. Every single pound of excess weight on your body puts 4 pounds of added stress on your knees. Over time, this extra burden on the knees can affect all of your weightbearing joints.

Many people do not realize is that obesity has an additional effect on your knee joints. Research shows that being obese stimulates a general increase in inflammation in the body, which can easily aggravate arthritic knees. It can cause or worsen knee pain day to day, and can make flare-ups last longer.

We must emphasize that obesity is a MAJOR risk factor for the development and progression of OA. Therefore, we ask patients with OA to consider getting their BMI below 30. Obesity is a medical diagnosis because it impacts more than just OA. Heart disease, diabetes, strokes, cancers, etc. are all influenced by obesity. Your weight loss efforts will provide benefits far beyond your joints.

BODY MASS INDEX CHART

Weight (pounds)

Height (feet & inches)	90	100	110	120	130	140	150	160	170	180	190	200	210	220	230	240	250	260
4' 10"	19	21	23	25	27	29	31	34	36	38	40	42	44	46	48	50	52	54
4' 11"	18	20	22	24	26	28	30	32	34	36	38	40	42	44	46	48	51	53
5'	18	20	22	23	25	27	29	31	33	35	37	39	41	43	45	47	49	51
5' 1"	17	19	21	23	25	26	28	30	32	34	36	38	40	42	44	45	48	50
5' 2"	17	18	20	22	24	26	27	29	31	33	35	37	38	40	42	44	46	48
5' 3"	16	18	20	21	23	25	27	28	30	32	34	35	37	39	41	43	44	46
5' 4"	15	17	19	21	22	24	26	28	29	31	33	34	36	38	40	41	43	45
5' 5"	15	17	18	20	22	23	25	27	28	30	32	33	35	37	38	40	43	45
5' 6"	15	16	18	19	21	23	24	26	27	29	31	32	34	36	37	39	40	42
5' 7"	14	16	17	19	20	22	24	25	27	28	30	31	33	35	36	38	39	41
5' 8"	14	15	17	18	20	21	23	24	26	27	29	30	32	34	35	37	38	40
5' 9"	13	15	16	18	19	21	22	24	25	27	28	30	31	33	34	35	37	38
5' 10"	13	14	16	17	19	20	22	23	24	26	27	29	30	32	33	34	36	37
5' 11"	13	14	15	17	18	20	21	22	24	25	26	28	29	31	32	33	35	36
6'	13	14	15	16	18	19	20	22	23	24	26	27	28	30	31	33	34	35
6' 1"	12	13	15	16	17	18	20	21	22	24	25	26	28	29	30	32	33	34
6' 2"	12	13	14	15	17	18	19	21	22	23	24	26	27	28	30	31	32	33
6' 3"	11	13	14	15	16	17	19	20	21	22	24	25	26	27	29	30	31	32
6' 4"	11	12	13	15	16	17	18	20	21	22	23	24	26	27	28	29	30	32
6' 5"	11	12	13	14	15	17	18	19	20	21	23	24	25	26	27	28	30	31
6' 6"	10	12	13	14	15	16	17	19	20	21	22	23	24	25	27	28	29	30

Underweight   Normal   Overweight   Obese

Directions for use: connect your weight and height to find your BMI number. If your BMI is 30+, you are in the category of obese, which is a major risk factor for osteoarthritis.

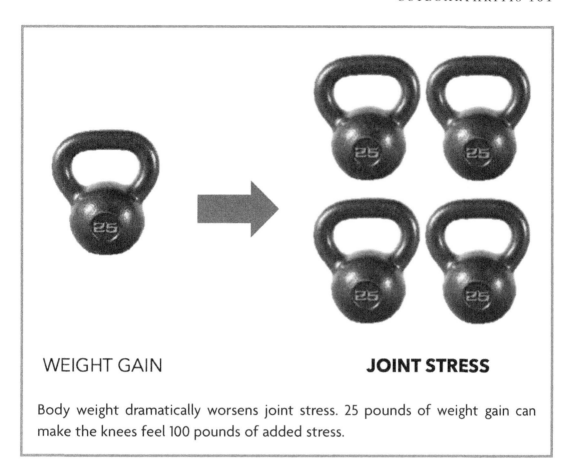

WEIGHT GAIN   **JOINT STRESS**

Body weight dramatically worsens joint stress. 25 pounds of weight gain can make the knees feel 100 pounds of added stress.

How can I lose weight if my knee pain won't allow me to exercise?

Weight loss is a challenge in general. But when arthritic patients are told to lose weight, they feel it is impossible because they feel they cannot exercise enough because of their knee pain. But fortunately, exercise is NOT required for successful weight loss, especially with OA. In fact, exercise on its own is not that efficient for losing weight. It can take 60+ minutes of exercise to burn 200 calories, which is time-consuming and laborious, and especially difficult/impossible on arthritic knees. However, a simple food substitution like eating an apple instead of a candy bar will eliminate 200 calories without any physical effort! Rather than spending 20 hours of exercise in a month hoping to burn the equivalent of 1 pound of weight, you can just skip 7 to 10 days of desserts!

Diet should always be the first step in a plan to lose weight. In fact, studies have shown that calorie restrictions are what make most weight loss programs succeed. Exercise is a good add-on that speeds up your metabolism to help make your diet more effective. But you really only need to do light, low impact of activities a few days a week to supplement your weight loss diet.

This is not the time in your life where you can literally muscle your way to weight loss, because your knees (and other joints) will not be up to the task of exercising enough to burn the required number of calories. Later we will discuss some low impact exercises that you can try in small doses, to maintain fitness and keep your metabolism running efficiently for better health.

I have tried losing weight so many times but it never works. What's the use?

Don't give up. Learn lessons from your past weight loss efforts, and try again. Some people have trouble losing weight, while others have trouble maintaining weight loss. If you were successful in losing weight but gained it back, at least you know that the weight can come off. If you have never been able to lose weight despite your best efforts, then perhaps you were trying too many gimmicks, or you need to consult with a nutritionist for help. In any case, you can always discuss this with your primary care doctor or endocrinologist to see if there is a medical reason preventing you from losing weight.

Use the power of positive thinking to help keep you disciplined and focused in a dedicated weight loss effort. We often tend to give up too easily without giving diet changes enough time to work, and negative thoughts are simply going to sabotage your efforts. Here are some diet tips to consider.

MAKE A MODEST GOAL: The ideal goal for weight loss is to get your BMI under 30, which is the threshold of obesity. Your current BMI may reveal that you have to lose a large amount of weight to get there, and this can feel overwhelming. But don't worry about losing the weight all at once. Make small manageable diet changes, and give yourself 3 months to lose the first 5 to 10 pounds. Repeat with similar goals every few months, and see how far you can get.

START WITH CALORIE CONTROL: The biggest factor in weight gain is a lack of calorie control. No matter what we eat, we seem to eat too much of it! To lose weight, you do not have to completely overhaul your diet. Simply start by eating less of each food item on your plate. For example, let's say you normally eat a 500 calorie serving of French fries with your lunch. Switch to a 200-calorie serving of small fries and save as much as 300 calories. You could also substitute for lower calorie foods whenever possible. If you eat a 150-calorie baked potato instead of those large fries, then you save 350 calories! You can make similar substitutions all day, every day. Another very easy example is to drink more water and less soda or other sugary drinks.

EAT SLOWLY! We pack in a lot of calories because we have a tendency to eat way too fast. Scientific studies show that after about 20-30 minutes your brain loses interest in eating and starts to feel full, dramatically decreasing your appetite. If you can slow down your eating past that 20-minute threshold, chances are good that you will eat less!

SEE A DIETITIAN: A dietitian is a certified meal advisor who can give you a customized, organized plan to lose weight. You will start with an analysis of your current diet pattern, calorie intake, and nutrition quality. Based on the evaluation, combined with your goals, you will get dietary recommendations built especially for you. It is important to realize that your community may have nutritionists, who are different than dietitians. Although guidelines vary from state to state in USA, nutritionists typically do not have specific certification but simply claim to be experts in giving nutritional advice.

GIVE IT TIME: Everyone looks for super-fast results when dieting, but it takes time for meaningful weight loss to occur. We gain weight over years or even decades. It is unreasonable to expect to lose it all in days or weeks. Diet programs that promise fast results often use extreme techniques that are too difficult to maintain. These diets will likely only have temporary benefits. Also, these diets can be unhealthy, making you feel terrible. The safest weight loss goes back to the basics, slow and steady. Realistically, a sensible plan will take

12 weeks to begin to see results. Then, give yourself 1-2 years to reach your desired target weight.

FOLLOW UP WITH YOUR DOCTOR: While you are in the process of losing weight, inform your doctor so that he/she can monitor your efforts and help guide you.

OK. I lost weight. Why do I still have pain?

Studies show that weight loss will reduce joint stress, and can help decrease pain. However, the effects may not be immediate, and there may only be partial relief. Also, your joints may need a lot of time for stress reduction to translate into pain relief. In some cases, the damage that is already done may be severe and weight loss may not be enough. You may also need to reduce other risk factors, modify your activities, get medical treatments, etc.

LIFESTYLE INTERVENTION 3: EAT HEALTHY FOODS

Besides weight loss, how else can food selection help someone with osteoarthritis(OA)?

We already discussed that weight loss for obese patients can help certain patients with OA. But diets should not just be designed for losing weight. A healthy diet focused on nutrition has additional benefits. Essentially, you can use food with high nutritional content as "natural medicine" to make your body function better. You can improve your energy, mood, and well-being while preventing illness and disease. For OA, healthy food choices can dramatically reduce painful inflammation.

What foods are good for OA?

Foods helpful for OA have nutrients that relieve painful inflammation. This anti-inflammatory effect may generally assist with healing and recovery for various musculoskeletal issues.

Fruits and veggies are the foundation of a healthy diet. For OA, most will have plenty of nutrients such as antioxidants that fight inflammation. Aim for a

MINIMUM of 5+ servings of fruits and veggies per day. You can refer to the table to see some specific items known to be particularly effective. Be aware that certain foods, even if considered healthy, may interact with medications you may be taking. Talk to your doctor whenever you make changes in your diet. .

Other foods with anti-inflammatory benefits include:
- Ginger
- Garlic
- Olive oil
- Turmeric
- Chia seeds
- Green tea

You should add these foods into your daily diet whenever you can. When you are very physically active, or if your OA flares up, then you should boost your anti-inflammatory food intake.

Antiinflammatory Diet Tips

1. Make healthy substitutions whenever possible.
2. Aim for 5-10 servings of fruits/veggies daily.
3. Mix fruits + veggies into juices and smoothies.
4. Boost your anti-inflammatory diet when you are more active or are starting to have pain.
5. Discuss all dietary changes with your doctor.

Special Antiinflammatory Foods

Fruits and Veggies	Other foods
• Dark green/leafy	• Whole grains
Kale, asparagus, spinach	*Breads, cereals, pasta*
• Bright colored	• Fish
Pineapple, carrots, berries	*Salmon, mackerel, trout*
• Olives	• Tea
Olives, olive oil	*Green tea*
• Pomegranates, Bing cherries	• Spices
Seasonal	*Turmeric, ginger*
• Cruciferous Veggies	• Nuts
Broccoli, Brussels sprouts	*Tree nuts (walnuts)*

LIFESTYLE INTERVENTION 4: AVOID UNHEALTHY FOODS

Are there foods that are bad for osteoarthritis(OA)?

Yes! There are foods that have been shown to trigger or aggravate inflammation in arthritic joints. Here are some examples:

Processed foods with refined carbohydrates are high in sugars, which promote inflammation. Refined grains (wheat), white rice, and cereals have been stripped of anti-inflammatory fibers and nutrients in the refining process. The foods containing refined carbohydrates are also filled with lots of chemicals and preservatives. These foods are everywhere, dressed up as boxed/prepackaged cookies and snacks. They fuel the production of chemicals in our body that trigger inflammation. Whole grain versions of grains, rice, and cereals are much healthier.

Desserts have several inflammatory ingredients that are a literal recipe for disaster for the joints. They tend to be high in sugars and saturated fats, which both increase inflammation. If they contain partially hydrogenated vegetable oils, then they are especially dangerous.

Sugary drinks are among the unhealthiest components of the American diet. The sugars, of course, are directly harmful. They are also high in calories, indirectly promoting obesity.

Fried foods are high in proinflammatory saturated fats. Most of the time, these foods are cooked in vegetable oils that have excessive omega-6 fats, which are also bad for the joints.

Red meat has been getting a lot of attention lately for possibly being generally unhealthy. We do know that when it comes to OA, there is a particular inflammatory chemical in red meat shown to increase inflammation in our bodies that could aggravate arthritic joints.

Nitrites also can stimulate increases in inflammation in the body that can affect the joints. Used as a preservative, these chemicals are found in various types of cured meats, and should be avoided.

Drinks that contain caffeine or alcohol may trigger increases in painful inflammation.

Allergenic foods contain certain chemicals that the body sees as unwelcome "foreign substances". This stimulates inflammatory responses in some people, causing widespread problems in the body. Common substances include glutens and artificial sweeteners.

Inflammatory Foods to Avoid with Osteoarthritis

1. Red meat
2. Fried foods
3. Sugary snacks
4. Refined grains (processed)
5. Alcohol/caffeine

LIFESTYLE INTERVENTION 5: REST!

How does "rest" help for osteoarthritis(OA)?

Knees with OA lack proper cushioning. They are not as durable as normal knees, and simply cannot put up with a lot of impact. Activity done in excess of what your knees can handle will cause a buildup of pain. Once the knees get aggravated past a certain point, the pain can last days or weeks. Therefore, rest is essential to nurture arthritic knees to promote recovery, avoiding a buildup of joint stress and inflammation when you are consistently active.

The first step is to be cautious during each strenuous activity or busy day. If you know you are going to be on your feet for a prolonged time period, take frequent breaks. Even if the activity does not seem that challenging, a 15-minute rest break will make a world of difference in reenergizing your knees. During a long day, offload your knees at every opportunity. For instance, during idle time when you have a choice to sit or stand, definitely sit down!

If you are generally busy every day, or you have an upcoming "busy time period" like a multiday vacation, pace yourself! Put limits on how much you are on your feet day to day. Always take at least one day off from physical activity per week as a rule. Don't wait for pain to slow you down—try to be proactive and take your breaks before trouble starts. And let's not forget about sleep…

> **Tips for Daytime Rest**
> - Take 5-10 minute breaks every hour to put your feet up.
> - Divide daily tasks into AM/PM sessions with rest in between.
> - Spread activities through the week instead of all in one day.
> - Do errands at off peak hours on off peak days to avoid lines.

Why is sleep important for osteoarthritis (OA)?

Sleep is a component of rest that is a very important part of all aspects of your general health. This are specific benefits for knee OA. Your body uses sleep for building and repairing body tissues. Sleep can help maintain healthy knees, and can help get rid of pain when OA flares up. Sleep is a simple intervention that could give arthritic knees better durability, faster recovery, and more mileage.

A good night of sleep has two necessary features: **quality and quantity.**

Quantity means that you get enough sleep time in a given day. There is no magic number of hours of sleep that are needed for good health. We use an average number of 7 to 8 hours per night, but individually, our bodies have unique needs. Some people need more sleep, while others seem to get by with much less. If you are always sleepy during the day, then you are definitely not getting enough sleep and should increase until you feel you can get through the day with better energy. If you are unsure, try to increase your nightly sleep average by 30 to 60 minutes for a month and check to see how much better you feel.

Quality means that your sleep session is restful and uninterrupted. Long stretches of quiet sleep have the best health benefits, as opposed to a choppy night of tossing and turning. A quiet, comfortable sleeping environment is essential! It is okay to take short naps through the day, if they don't interfere with your ability to get a full night's sleep through the night.

You can review the tips on the following page to help you with both quality and quantity to get the best out of your sleep. If you are having persistent issues with fatigue or a lack of energy, especially if you have already improved your sleep habits, follow up with your primary care physician to see if there may be a medical cause.

Tips for better sleep

1. Aim for better QUANTITY.
- Prioritize sleep.
  Cut nonessential activities like TV or reading, to get to bed earlier.

- Go to bed at the same time at night.
  Research suggests the best quality of sleep will be between 10 pm and 6 am.

- Don't read, eat, or watch TV in bed.
  Avoid late night screentime that may interfere with your ability to fall asleep.

- Exercise early!
  Vigorous exercise too late in the day can interfere with nighttime sleepiness.

- Aim for daily consistency.
  Don't wait for the weekend to "catch up"- get enough sleep every night.

2. Aim for better QUALITY.
- Avoid caffeine.
  Daytime caffeine intake can make it difficult to fall or stay asleep.

- Stop smoking.
  Smoking can create nighttime withdrawal symptoms, causing restless sleep.

- Eat dinner early.
  Eat early enough to get a few hours of "digestion time" before sleep.

- Exercise early.
  Vigorous exercise too late in the day could also lead to restless sleep.

- Keep room temperature comfortable.
  Avoid struggling through the night because of a room that is too hot/cold.

CHAPTER 6
ACTIVITY MODIFICATIONS

Many people with knee osteoarthritis are physically active and want to stay that way. If you are in this category, you may have lots of questions about what you should and should not be doing. This section will teach you how to make appropriate changes to stay on your feet in a way that protects your joints.

Is physical activity good or bad for osteoarthritis(OA)?

Exercise has wide ranging benefits for your overall health, and for your general well-being. Regular exercise, when done properly, is good for knees with OA. Physical activity helps maintain muscle strength that supports aging knee joints for daily tasks. But with knee OA, your joints have limits. They are delicate and vulnerable to inflammation and injury. Exercise must be approached with great caution to prevent overuse, so that you get all the health benefits of exercise without causing further damage to your joints.

I thought I am supposed to be exercising 30 minutes every day.

Exercise guidelines that you hear from different agencies and organizations are for the general population. In reality, each individual has his/her limits, depending on age, health status, etc. Your goal for exercise should be to do enough to get the benefits, but not to the point where there are risks to the body. With osteoarthritis, the joints have durability up to a point, and it is important to respect this limit.

My doctor did tell me that I am overdoing it, but I have been doing the same workouts successfully for the past 10 years—why do I have to change now?

Just because a workout schedule or routine worked for the past 10 years doesn't mean it will be good for you forever! Our bodies are constantly changing, and we must factor in the natural aging process in our exercise planning. As we get older, our bodies will heal more slowly and get injured more easily. The "wear and tear" process can accelerate with age, and we should pay close attention to how our muscles, bones, and joints are responding to our daily schedules.

It's impossible for your doctor to know how much exercise is too much, because everyone is different. If you are starting to experience knee pain, then you should take an honest look at your exercise regimen. Make reasonable changes that protect your joints. Find a "new normal" with a new activity schedule that properly takes into account the limitations of arthritic knees.

How do I know if I need to change my physical activities?

When you have osteoarthritis, knee pain should provoke you to consider making activity modifications. Especially if there wasn't a particular injury, pain indicates that you are simply doing more than what your knees can handle. Start by modifying the activity that you think is most directly causing your knee pain. If you are unsure, then make changes across the board at work and/or at home, sports/hobbies, etc.

What activities should I quit?

High impact activities cause excessive stress in arthritic knees. These are the sports and hobbies that require running, jumping, repetitive twisting, kneeling, squatting, and/or pivoting. Other activities that involve sudden unpredictable movements, falls, and collisions should also be retired.

I only do light exercise. Do I need to make changes in my schedule?

All activities can become dangerous when you do more than what your body can handle. People often think, *"I'm just walking so I can do it as much as I want*", but stress builds up in the joints even with low impact activities done too aggressively. If you are getting knee pain, then yes, you may need to make some changes even for "light" exercise.

How do I modify my physical activities?

There are 3 main ways to change your activities to make them safer for your knees:

1. Modify the intensity (the amount of exertion) of the activity.
2. Modify the duration (minutes per session) of the activity.
3. Modify the frequency (days per week) of the activity.

If you are having knee pain, then try one or more of these modifications until you find a "new normal" that allows you to be active symptom-free.

- **Modify INTENSITY**: avoid going "all out" when you exercise. Take the edge off and exercise at a more leisurely pace that allows you to maintain a level of comfort from beginning to end. Simply enjoy the moment! Choose slower speeds, avoid hills and rough terrain, etc. If you like challenges and insist on pushing yourself, do yourself a favor and alternate easy, medium, and hard days to avoid constantly redlining every time you exercise.

- **Modify DURATION**: Consider cutting your exercise times to minimize joint stress and improve recovery. For example, we are programmed to think that we should exercise for an hour. In fact, group classes and training sessions, even for seniors, are routinely scheduled for 60 minutes. Avoid falling into the "one hour" trap and adjust your participation to suit your needs. Depending on the exercise, you may only need 15 minute sessions or less to get the health benefits of physical activity. For group sessions, simply sit out part of the class, or you can talk to your fitness instructor about giving you a shorter workout.

Exercising with a friend is great for motivation and camaraderie. However, when 2 people are at different levels of fitness, one will be doing too much when they work out together. Avoid the pressure of joining a friend's 90 minute walk when you know your knees realistically can only handle 45 minutes.

If you are dealing with ongoing mild pain or a new flare-up, you may need to cut the duration of all workouts by 50 to 75% until you are feeling better. Once you recover, consider new time limits to keep your knees healthy.

- **Modify FREQUENCY**: Always take at least 1-2 days off per week from vigorous exercise. Your body needs more rest as you get older, for proper repair and recovery. Also, avoid doing two different strenuous activities in the same day. Overlapping activities will easily overwhelm your knees, especially if they both require a lot of leg impact.

ACTIVITY QUESTIONNAIRE
Are you at risk for overuse?
Too much activity will aggravate arthritic knees

Fill in the following chart with your typical weekly activities:

ACTIVITY	MINUTES/ SESSION	DAYS PER WEEK (CIRCLE)	DID YOUR KNEE PAIN STOP THIS ACTIVITY?
		S S M T W R F	☐YES ☐NO
		S S M T W R F	☐YES ☐NO
		S S M T W R F	☐YES ☐NO
		S S M T W R F	☐YES ☐NO
		S S M T W R F	☐YES ☐NO
		S S M T W R F	☐YES ☐NO

Examine your schedule above. Look for signs of overuse:
1. Too many activities in the same day.
2. Too much total time spent exercising in a given day.
3. Too many total activities per week.
4. Less than 1 day of complete rest per week.

Be proactive to protect arthritic joints:
1. Respect your knee's limits.
2. Make changes in your schedule until you can be active without pain.

What if I enjoy hard workouts?

The "go hard or go home" mentality will eventually lead to early retirement from your activities. When pushed to the limit, your muscles get fatigued, and your form and coordination quickly deteriorate. This can lead to dramatic increases in joint stress, putting your knees at risk for painful inflammation or major injury. Tough workouts may feel invigorating, but they are risky and can speed up the "wear and tear" in arthritic knees. Constantly "going for it" can cause you to literally run your knees into the ground, especially as you get older. Exercise is considered healthy, but is harmful when done in extremes!

I participate in multiple different activities through the week. Can I continue?

Doing several activities a week can be good because variation could round out your fitness while preventing overuse. However, some issues may occur when you pack too many activities into your daily schedule. Multiple exercise sessions done too close together will risk overuse. Avoid overlap as much as possible: Limit yourself to one activity per day.

- Take at least one day totally off from strenuous exercise per week.
- Avoid multiple activities where you are using the same muscles/movements.

You may not even realize how much you are doing over the course of a week. The activity questionnaire above will help analyze your weekly schedule for overuse.

What about my dog that needs longer walks?

Don't worry- you can make modifications to keep your dog happy without wearing out your joints. You may have to use one of the dog's walks as your main exercise session for the day. When going out for walks, choose pathways with secure footing. Look for even terrain that avoids hills. For active dogs that need more exercise than you can handle, there are several options. If you have a controlled environment like a fenced in yard, then you can play fetch to get your dog to run around while you stay put. Also, if you have a reasonably safe dog park nearby, drive there and let your dog burn through his/her energy quota while you relax. For a dog that needs multiple outings, get the rest of your family involved to share the dog walking responsibilities!

How should I handle new activities?

Perhaps you are active and you are thinking of a new sport or hobby to keep life interesting. Or, maybe you are trying to start exercising consistently. Either scenario can easily overload arthritic knees. Therefore, any change in your activity level has to be approached with care. Please abide by the following rules to minimize your osteoarthritis (OA) risk:

1. **Start small.** ALWAYS introduce new activities slowly. Start with 10-15 minute mini-sessions for a few weeks to get your muscles and joints loosened up and accustomed to new movement patterns. Don't forget that your heart and lungs also need time to get properly conditioned. Stick with light, short duration sessions for 4 weeks. After that, if your body feels OK, then you can consider increasing each workout by 5-10 minutes.

2. **Allow time for rest.** Limit new activities to 2 times a week, with a few days of space in between, to see how your body responds. It takes time to know for sure if you can handle the new activity at its current level.

3. **Low impact only.** Never start or resume a high-impact, high-risk sport. At your age, your body/knees will never hold up to relentless pounding, falling, twisting, pivoting, etc. Be smart! Choose activities that will add to your fitness without causing or increasing bodily damage.

4. **Watch for warning signs.** Pain during an activity is a red flag indicating that you should immediately stop what you are doing. Any soreness after a new activity that does not disappear within a day could quickly develop into a much bigger problem. Joint swelling, gradual or sudden, is always indicative of a problem. Also, fatigue, cramps, restlessness, numbness/tingling, weakness are all symptoms that should never be ignored. Always seek medical guidance for symptoms you develop with exercise.

5. **Don't start training for marathons!** Choose activities that make sense for what your knees can realistically handle. Realize that this is no longer the time to start chasing ambitious exercise goals you should have set when you were 20 years old. Also, avoid coming out of retirement for high-risk activities you enjoyed in the past. There is often a reason you left an activity in the rearview years ago.

How do shoes affect my activities?

For light or casual daily activities of short duration, your footwear may not matter. However, for dedicated exercise, labor work, and prolonged physical activity, choosing the appropriate shoes can make a huge difference for keeping your knees healthy. A good pair of shoes will help maintain leg alignment, prevent injuries, and absorb forces from the ground. First, always wear shoes made specifically for a given activity. Shoes should fit your foot in length and width, and should have good support and traction. The shoe should be built with plenty of cushioning and support. Cushioning is important for shock absorption, and stability and stiffness provide support important for proper biomechanics. Don't forget to change your "activity" shoes every 6 to 9 months or sooner.

How does my job impact my knees?

Many people have labor-intensive occupations that can cause injuries and joint stress similar to a sport. Frequent bending/kneeling/squatting/pivoting and constant repetitive movements are particularly bad. Some jobs involve high-risk activities that lead to frequent accidents, which could cause or worsen knee osteoarthritis.

Meanwhile, even a desk job can also be painful for arthritic knees, depending on your workstation and the number of hours you are in a stationary sitting position.

How can I protect my knees at work?

If you have knee osteoarthritis and you are still working, then you should evaluate your job duties and workstation. Make whatever changes you can to protect your joints. Try to negotiate with your employer to implement long-term work modifications. If you see writing on the wall that your knees simply cannot handle your workload, then consider a career move to a less physical position.

- **Modify!** Whether you are a heavy laborer or office worker, you may be doing repetitive activities that are harmful to your knees. Obviously, heavy lifting, crawling, climbing, etc. in physical careers like construction and plumbing are stressful to your joints. But keep in mind that any pivoting, turning, bending, and kneeling, even in an office setting, can aggravate arthritic knees. Ask your doctor for a note recommending reasonable work modifications and take it to your employer.

- **Sit!** If you have a job that requires you to stand or walk for long periods of time, consider asking for longer or more frequent breaks so that you can give your knees some rest. If you are stationed in a standing position at work, then ask for a stool or chair. Stretch regularly to keep your muscles loose and functional.

- **Stand!** Whether you are a driver or have a desk job, jobs that require sitting all day can make your knees stiff and painful from being in one position for prolonged time. Plan mini-breaks to stand up and walk around.

- **Adjust your workstation!** People may think that their sit-down area at work only affects their neck, back, and arms. However, your seating position can aggravate your knees whether or not you have osteoarthritis. Ask your employer for an ergonomic evaluation, where an expert visits your work area and recommends adjustments that will take stress off your joints. Depending on your job, this may require changes in desk height, chair, driver's seat position, etc.

- **Change jobs or retire!** Strenuous occupations like construction or plumbing put unavoidable stress on your knees over a lifetime. Such careers simply are not sustainable for healthy knees. Always be on the lookout for a less physically demanding job position. Supervisor roles may dramatically decrease physical work. In any case, consider what's available, including retirement.

- **Find support!** There are many ways to support your knees through hectic workdays.
  - Bring healthy meals and snacks with you to keep the inflammation away.
  - As much as possible, wear comfortable, supportive shoes at work and/or during your commute.
  - Talk to your doctor about a knee brace for support during any physical work that you do.

What if I have specific questions about my activities?

We have given you general guidelines so you have a basic understanding of options that can help you. If you need specific recommendations about your daily routine and exercise schedule, make an appointment to see a physical therapist or sports doctor. Either health professional can give you advice to personalize changes in your activities.

CHAPTER 7
MEDICAL TREATMENTS

So far we have discussed lifestyle modifications to give you long-term strategies to help manage your osteoarthritis (OA). There are several medical interventions that can help you as well. Many are designed for pain relief, which can be used for both short and long term interventions for your OA. Your doctor may prescribe treatment and/or give you options for medical self-help remedies that can be done at home.

What are the basic medical options that my doctor can recommend?

There are several medical treatment options, depending on your short term needs and long term goals. These treatments include:

- **Oral medications** such as anti-inflammatories, narcotic tablets, and chronic pain modulators can help control pain.
- **Topical relievers** like capsaicin, salicylates, menthol and lidocaine can soothe achy knees.
- **Knee injections** can reduce pain and improve function.
- **Physical therapy** has been proven to improve function and decrease arthritis pain over time.
- **Assistive devices** like knee braces, canes and walkers can provide knee support and pain relief.
- **Regenerative treatments** claim to preserve or rebuild cartilage but are unproven.

- **Surgery** is a big step but may offer relief for severe osteoarthritis when conservative measures have failed.

What is the goal of medical treatments?

Your doctor will help you achieve an overall goal to improve or maintain your quality of life despite your osteoarthritis (OA). Medical treatments can reduce or eliminate pain to keep you physically active. Interventions like physical therapy may also improve function and durability over time. A well-constructed plan of action that includes medical intervention could possibly slow the progression of the "wear and tear".

MEDICAL TREATMENT 1: HOME TREATMENTS

What doctor-recommended medical treatments can I try at home?

1. Both ice and heat have been shown to have benefits for pain relief with osteoarthritis (OA). Both are relatively safe, but should be used with caution:

   - **Ice** may help relieve OA pain by decreasing inflammation in and around the knee. Ice can be used up to 3 to 4 times a day as needed for pain flare-ups, and after physical activity. You can buy or make an ice pack, or grab something like a bag of frozen vegetables from the freezer. Ice is applied to sore areas around the joint in short time intervals.

     Although it is a good therapeutic intervention, ice should be used with caution. Continuous use can irritate, aggravate, and permanently injure body tissue. For specific instructions, ask your doctor or therapist.

   - **Heat** may help soothe and relieve pain in arthritic knees, and may reduce stiffness. A heating pad or warm moist towel can be recommended for a few minutes at a time a few times a day, but you must be careful not to burn your skin. For specific instructions, discuss with your doctor or physical therapist.

2. **A simple knee sleeve or wrap** may make your knee feel better or more secure. The compression effects can also help control swelling. You can buy them online or at a local pharmacy, most of the time without a prescription. Knee sleeves come in all shapes and sizes, so you may have to try a few variations to find one that fits and works best for you. If a sleeve/wrap is too tight, or if you have problems with your circulation, then you have to use caution otherwise you could develop leg swelling, rashes, numbness, or skin breakdown. Talk to your doctor.

3. **Over the counter medications** like acetaminophen (pain reliever) and anti-inflammatories such as ibuprofen or naproxen may be useful for occasional mild knee pain. You can get them without a prescription, but let your doctor know before using them. Over the counter medications are as strong as prescriptions. They can cause or aggravate liver, kidney, lung, or digestive problems, and can trigger severe allergic reactions.

MEDICAL TREATMENT 2: PRESCRIPTION MEDICATIONS

How do anti-inflammatory medications help for osteoarthritis (OA)?

Anti-inflammatory medications can improve OA symptoms of pain, swelling, and stiffness. They are administered by mouth in pill or capsule form, and there are topical versions as well. Although there are a couple of over the counter options, most have to be prescribed by a physician.

These medications can be used as needed for pain for short durations of time, although some doctors prescribe them to be taken daily. Although they are considered reasonably safe medications, they can have numerous side effects. These include serious conditions such as heart disease, permanent kidney damage, bleeding in the digestive tract, and swelling. They can also aggravate conditions such as hypertension and asthma. Some people may have severe allergic reactions that can be life-threatening. Antiinflammatory medications may interact with other medications you are taking, so check with your doctor and pharmacist.

Can I take pain medications for OA?

There are several different types of pain medications. They do not have any direct effect in treating the causes of OA. These are purely symptom relievers that should only be taken when you feel you absolutely need them, and should not be used routinely on a schedule "just in case". They are mostly tablets and capsules, but can be given by injection.

Acetaminophen (popular brand name TYLENOL) is an over the counter medication that is very useful for OA. It is purely a pain reliever for various mild to moderate aches, including osteoarthritis, with no anti-inflammatory properties. It can be used to manage flare-ups that interfere with normal daily activities or sleep. Acetaminophen can affect the liver or kidneys, but in normal therapeutic doses should be relatively safe for healthy people.

Narcotics encompass a broad class of powerful pain medications that effectively block pain receptors in your brain for dramatic relief of symptoms. They can only be acquired legally with a prescription. There are several types of narcotics of varying strengths. They are prescribed individually or in combination with acetaminophen.

Narcotic treatments can be very complex. There are different regimens and combinations. Narcotics have serious effects on the body. They are addictive and commonly abused. Therefore, anyone taking narcotics long-term should be closely monitored by a physician. Once you start taking these medications for chronic pain, it is very difficult to stop.

What are neuromodulators?

Pain modulators range from antidepressants to seizure medications that have been found to be effective for patients with chronic pain syndromes. They are not approved by the FDA to specifically treat osteoarthritis. They tend to adjust your body's response to pain to take the edge off of constant symptoms, but they do not treat arthritis in any way. They are not considered first line medications for osteoarthritis. However, for ongoing pain otherwise difficult to control, they could be an option that your doctors could discuss with you. These medications must be taken consistently to build up to the point where they will work. They cannot be taken only as needed for sudden increases in pain. They are usually started slowly to allow the body to become accustomed to taking them As a result, it could take weeks or months to find out if they work for you. Each has its own specific side effect profile, and can interact with other medications that you may be taking.

What topicals can I use for osteoarthritis (OA)?

There are many over the counter topical gels, creams, and lotions that you can rub on your joints that may help relieve knee pain. Depending on the active ingredient, they work in different ways to soothe achy joints. Even though they generally have low side effect profiles, always discuss with your doctor before trying any topical preparation. Also, remember that ice is a very safe and effective topical treatment that is medication-free!

These days, there has been a sudden rush of advertising for cannabidiol (CBD)-based topicals derived from hemp or marijuana plants for knee pain. To date, they have not been scientifically proven to work for relieving osteoarthritis symptoms.

MEDICAL TREATMENT 3: INJECTIONS

What does a "cortisone" injection do?

"Cortisone" is the popular name for medications in the corticosteroid (steroid) family. Corticosteroids are powerful anti-inflammatory hormones used for many medical conditions. They can be administered orally as a tablet or by injection. Even though they are very effective in reducing inflammation quickly. corticosteroids have a long list of common side effects. For musculoskeletal conditions like knee OA, "cortisone" is rarely given in the oral form by specialists because it is safer and much more effective if it's injected directly into the joint.

"Cortisone" is injected into an arthritic joint to decrease inflammation during a flare up. It can temporarily relieve pain and swelling, but does not heal, "fix", or cure osteoarthritis.

Are "cortisone" injections safe?

Corticosteroids (also known as "cortisone" or steroid) are strong anti-inflammatory medications. When they are prescribed to be taken as tablets by mouth, corticosteroids have widespread effects throughout the body. Risks include weight gain, osteoporosis, avascular necrosis (bone death), mood changes, cataracts, and blood sugar changes. With joint injections, corticosteroids are supposedly less risky because it is thought that the medicine is confined to the joint with minimal spread to the rest of the body. However, short-term skin flushing and blood sugar changes are known to occur with injections, so there may be some risks of spread outside of the joint.

Steroid injections have a risk of joint infection (probably around 1 in 1000). Also, "cortisone" can have direct local effects that add to cartilage degeneration in the arthritic joint. Although the degenerative effects are probably small with a single injection, the risk increases when injections are repeated over time.

There is no established consensus on how "cortisone" joint injections should be administered. Each doctor will have a set preference in dosing, frequency and total number of "cortisone" knee injections for a given patient. For instance, you may hear that "cortisone" injections should not be given more than 3 times per joint in a lifetime. But in many cases, injections are given multiple times over many years. Some doctors think that "cortisone" injections should be discontinued if pain returns after one or two doses. The reality is that "cortisone" injections will not "fix", heal, or cure OA. However, they can provide temporary relief to help manage disruptive OA symptoms, which is an important treatment tool. Steroid injections are generally thought to be relatively safe if given in the same joint at least 3 to 6 months apart for knee OA. Adjustments in dosing and frequency are considered depending on age, coexisting health conditions, degree of OA, etc.

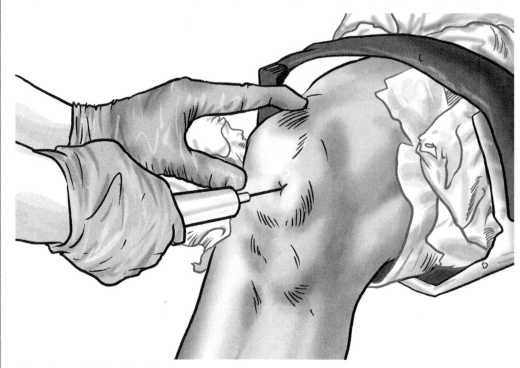

"Cortisone" injection (patient seated).

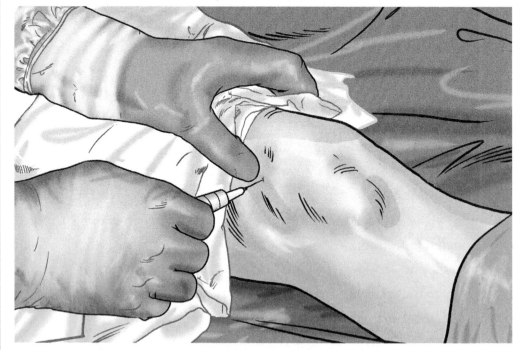

"Cortisone" injection (patient lying down).

When should I have a "cortisone" injection?

Because of the risks, especially for joint damage over time, "cortisone" injections should be avoided unless it is needed for a moderate to severe osteoarthritis pain flare-up that does not resolve with rest, icing, medications, and time.

How is a "cortisone" injection given?

A corticosteroid injection is given during a regular doctor's visit. You will either sit or lie down for the injection. The procedure is simple. Your doctor will clean the skin, then give the injection with a needle placed into the joint. If your knee is swollen, your doctor may insert a needle into the joint remove the fluid before administering the medication. Both knees can be injected in the same office visit. After the injection, you may be asked to rest from strenuous activities, but you will be able to walk out of the office and drive home. You should not have to miss work and you can continue your normal daily routine. The injection preparation usually contains a fast-acting numbing agent mixed with the "cortisone", so your knee may feel a bit better for a few hours. However, the "cortisone" often takes a few days to take effect.

"Cortisone" injections don't work because my pain keeps coming back- why?

"Cortisone" injections will not cure osteoarthritis. At best, they temporarily relieve pain by reducing inflammation for some period of time. If you get relief for 3 months or longer, the injection is considered a success, and can be repeated if needed at least 3 months apart.

When should I avoid having a "cortisone" injection?

- If you have not had x-rays, or if your x-rays are normal, then you may not have osteoarthritis. A "cortisone" injection should not be given until your diagnosis is confirmed.

- If you recently had a trauma, you may have torn, broken, or otherwise injured something in your knee. With this possibility, other treatments may be needed, and a steroid injection should not be given before a diagnosis is made.

- If you have uncontrolled diabetes, a "cortisone" injection could cause a catastrophic increase in your blood sugars so should be avoided.

- If you are having severe pain with an inability to move the knee or bear weight, you may have a problem other than OA and the "cortisone" injection can make your knee worse. In this scenario, you should immediately see a specialist for an evaluation.

- If your pain is mild, then you should try other less invasive treatments to save your knees unnecessary steroid exposure.

- You probably should not have an injection "just in case" when you are having little or no pain but want to try to prevent a flare-up before an event or vacation.

Do hyaluronic acid injections work?

Viscosupplementation injections with hyaluronic acid (HA) are FDA-approved for treatment of mild to moderate osteoarthritis. Patients often mistakenly refer to viscosupplementation treatment as "gel" or "lubricant" injections. HA is a chemical that is naturally produced by the body to nourish the knee joint by stimulating the production of important proteins. It is thought that having more HA in the knee may help protect cartilage and prevent osteoarthritis (OA) from getting worse.

Unfortunately, HA injections have not been definitively proven to be more effective than traditional treatments including "cortisone" injections for OA pain relief. However, according to patient testimonials, people do describe benefits of pain reduction for up to several months. Also, some patients feel that the HA injections make their knee(s) feel more durable and better able to handle their physical activities. There are the usual risks of infection because of the injection itself, and some people get temporary joint irritation called "synovitis" that can cause pain and swelling. Otherwise, the injections are largely regarded as safe.

What about PRP or stem cell injections for knee osteoarthritis (OA)?

Regenerative treatments use the body's own healing powers to relieve OA pain. The mechanisms of action of these emerging therapies are thought to range from anti- inflammatory effects to tissue rebuilding. They are currently used for many medical conditions.

Platelet-rich plasma (PRP) is found in our blood. In a concentrated form, PRP is thought to have special healing effects. PRP is extracted from a sample of your own blood, and then injected into the knee joint. PRP has been shown to have beneficial effects for various orthopedic conditions. However, the dose and frequency needed to make a difference are unknown. Also, research for PRP used specifically for knee OA is inconclusive so far.

Stem cell therapy is another type of regenerative treatment used for knee OA. The theory is that stem cells can reprogram themselves to build healthy tissue wherever they are placed. For OA, stem cells injected into a knee joint would ideally be able to replace and rebuild cartilage that has been lost or damaged in the degenerative process that leads to OA. But research has generated more questions than answers. Also, in USA, true stem cells from embryo and fetal tissue are not available. Instead, cells from our own bone marrow are extracted and used to treat OA. These are not true stem cells, are found in small amounts, and the effectiveness of bone marrow aspirates is highly questionable.

Unfortunately, these regenerative "cell therapy" treatments are expensive and unpredictable. There is some evidence that pain, swelling, and movement can improve with cell therapies, but research is far from perfect. Claims of cartilage regrowth and reversal of OA are always going to be difficult to prove. Nevertheless, some people searching for a "fix" that traditional medicine cannot provide will invariably gravitate to these treatments. There is no established protocol, so we don't even know how many injections to give, how often, etc. We also do not know how long a treatment will work, which is very concerning given the high cost per dose. Cell therapies are generally not covered by insurance. At some point, we may figure it all out. We are hoping that regenerative medicine may eventually become a "go-to" to save our joints. But at this time, we simply do not have enough convincing information.

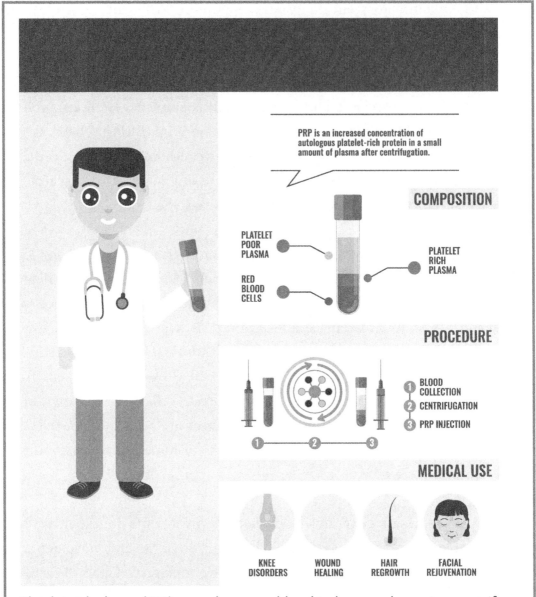

PRP is an increased concentration of autologous platelet-rich protein in a small amount of plasma after centrifugation.

COMPOSITION

PLATELET POOR PLASMA

RED BLOOD CELLS

PLATELET RICH PLASMA

PROCEDURE

1 BLOOD COLLECTION
2 CENTRIFUGATION
3 PRP INJECTION

MEDICAL USE

KNEE DISORDERS · WOUND HEALING · HAIR REGROWTH · FACIAL REJUVENATION

Platelet rich plasma (PRP) procedure: your blood is drawn and spun in a centrifuge to separate the PRP, which is then collected and injected into the area of concern.

MEDICAL TREATMENT 4: PHYSICAL THERAPY

How does physical therapy help people with osteoarthritis (OA)?

Physical therapy (PT) is considered a very important medical treatment for osteoarthritis. It has been shown to improve function, meaning people can move around better, with greater endurance and durability. Also, physical therapy may decrease pain episodes over the long term, and may prevent progression of OA.

A good physical therapy program for osteoarthritis will improve:

- **Flexibility:** Stretches will help prevent stiff joints and preserve movement.
- **Core stability:** A strong core gives you better body control to promote freedom and efficiency of leg movement.
- **Strength:** Leg strength protects and supports your knee joints while giving you better durability in your activities.
- **Balance:** Being steadier on your feet ensures efficient movement, decreases joint stress, and prevents falls.

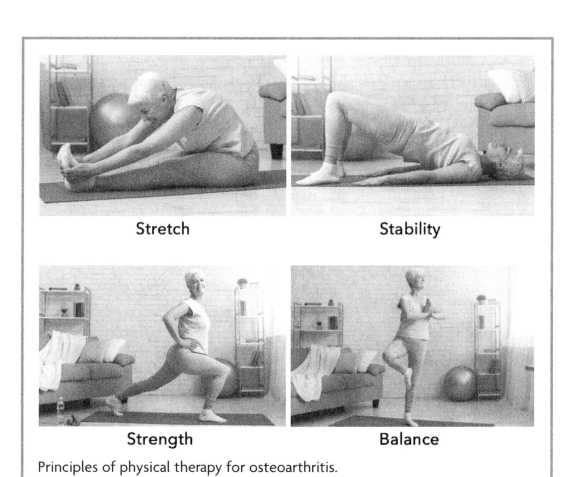

Stretch

Stability

Strength

Balance

Principles of physical therapy for osteoarthritis.

Do all patients with osteoarthritis need to go to physical therapy (PT)?

PT offers benefits for every type of patient with knee osteoarthritis. For people having a lot of knee pain, PT can focus on the basics for reducing inflammation and regaining leg function. For athletes with OA looking for an edge to keep them on the playing field, PT will emphasize advanced level protocols for better performance and injury prevention through agility, stability, coordination, and balance. Older, frail patients will get simple conditioning exercises to make normal daily activities easier, prevent falls, and maintain as much independence as possible.

What should I expect from physical therapy?

- Physical therapy can help you manage your OA pain and improve your function.
- Physical therapy can help you stay on your feet.
- Physical therapy is only one part of a comprehensive plan of care that you and your doctor create together that includes home care, activity modification, and medical treatment.
- Physical therapy requires occasional office visits, but it only works when you are an active participant in the prescribed home exercises you do between office sessions.
- Improvements in strength, stamina, balance, and flexibility can take at least 3 months to kick in, and will always require an ongoing maintenance process.

What WON'T physical therapy do?

- Physical therapy will not cure your knee osteoarthritis.
- Physical therapy cannot be expected to treat severe pain- this is a situation where you will need evaluation and other medical treatment from your knee specialist.
- Physical therapy will not fix you in one day. You can expect to have about 6 to 12 sessions, but you will have to work on your home program for months to get good results.

- Physical therapy cannot work if you don't put in the time and effort. It requires your active interest and participation.

Can't someone just give me the exercises so I can do them at home?

Physical therapy isn't "one size fits all". Ideally, each person gets a personalized rehabilitation program based on their specific goals and level of fitness. Your therapist performs an evaluation and recommends specific exercises based on observations of your individual deficits in strength, balance, core stability, and flexibility. If you do not have the option to see a therapist, then a handout of exercises are probably better than nothing. However, if seeing a therapist is an available resource, you should utilize it if you decide that you want to try and get maximum benefits of physical therapy.

MEDICAL TREATMENT 5: KNEE BRACES

Should I try a knee brace?

Research isn't overwhelmingly positive to support the use of knee bracing, but the American Association of Orthopedic Surgeons agrees that knee braces *may* be helpful for managing osteoarthritis. There are many different options. The braces are only helpful when you wear them, providing support, stability, or comfort during physical activity. A knee brace is a worthwhile option if you are looking for ways to help stay on your feet.

What types of braces are available?

- **"Unloader" braces** are specifically designed for knee osteoarthritis when there is decreased space in either side of the joint. These rigid, bulky plastic or carbon fiber braces put sideways pressure to increase the joint space and prevent the bones from rubbing together. They can be custom made and tuned to your specific needs. Your doctor has to prescribe this brace, and depending on your insurance, it can be expensive.

- **Velcro braces** are made from neoprene or similar thick, soft material. They come in all shapes and sizes, with many structural variations. They use adjustable straps, and may have metal hinges on the sides for better support. For patellar (kneecap) osteoarthritis, "patellofemoral" brace variations are available, with extra rubber support in the front to help maintain kneecap alignment. Some are available by prescription, but most can be purchased on your own.

- **Knee sleeves** are the most basic "all purpose" form of knee support, made with stretchy elastic that you simply pull up like a sock over the knee. Knee sleeves provide simple compression that can reduce swelling. The compressive fit tends to feel comforting or nurturing. However, sleeves lack hardware and therefore do not provide any true stabilizing support. They are inexpensive and can also be found in different sizes.

Talk to your doctor if you are interested in trying a knee brace. Custom braces must be prescribed, and are typically dispensed by brace companies or medical supply stores. Some orthopedic offices stock "off the shelf" braces and sleeves in their offices. Otherwise, you can ask where braces and sleeves can be purchased locally. In the general marketplace, they are usually available in pharmacies, sporting goods stores, and online.

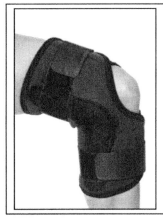

VELCRO BRACE

- Many varieties
- No prescription needed
- Adjustable velcro straps
- With or without metal hinge support
- May unload patella (kneecap)

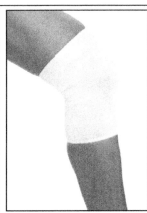

KNEE SLEEE

- Simple, inexpensive
- Lightweight
- Can control swelling
- No structural support
- "Nurturing comfort"

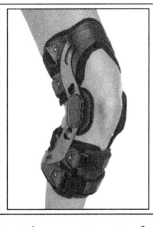

UNLOADER BRACE

- Custom made
- Must be prescribed/ordered by M.D.
- Structural support for physical activity
- Manually opens collapsed arthritic joint
- Bulky, heavy

Basic brace categories for osteoarthritis.

When should I use my brace?

You can use a brace during the day with physical activity when you feel that your knee needs support to get through your activities. You may choose to wear it only when you know you will be engaging in prolonged physical activity, or only when you are having pain. You may find the best results when you use a brace in conjunction with other assistive devices like canes/walkers.

I feel like I wasted money on a knee brace. Now what?

A knee brace is worth a try when you are looking for added support to keep you active in sports, hobbies, or independent living. Unfortunately, it is impossible to know which brace or sleeve will work for you because there are so many different types out there. Plus, everyone's situation is different. There are many variables such as body shape, amount of arthritis, and activity level that make brace selection mostly trial and error. Your doctor or therapist will be the best resources to increase your chances of finding a brace that meets your needs. However, there is always a chance that the brace you paid for won't work. You shouldn't let yourself get upset or frustrated. It is always ideal to try the brace on before buying it, if possible. As long as it is not increasing your pain, you should allow for some time to see if the brace eventually works or not—the effects are not always immediate. Also, even if it didn't provide miraculous benefits, see if there are at least some situations where the brace is useful before giving up on it entirely. Just because one brace doesn't work, you can still try another if you are still looking for knee support. Or, different braces may help in different situations. If and when you do find a good brace, it can keep you on your feet, relieve your pain, etc.

MEDICAL TREATMENT 6: ASSISTIVE DEVICES

Why are assistive devices helpful for osteoarthritis(OA)?

Assistive devices like canes, walkers, and wheelchairs are very useful for painful knee OA. When knee pain gets to the point where walking is bothersome most or all the time, assistive devices take the stress off your knee joints to help keep you moving with less pain. The use of an assistive device to offload the knee is a powerful tool for recovery when your knee flares up. Also, assistive devices prevent limping that causes overloading in other joints.

You can plan out when you want to use assistive devices. You may need one all the time, or only with prolonged time on your feet, or with certain activities, or only when there is extreme pain. You may choose to use different assistive devices depending on your schedule or situation on any given day.

Will a cane help me?

The cane is a very useful assistive device for active people with one painful knee. A cane effectively offloads the knee to improve your ability to stay mobile. You can use a cane as a preventive measure if you know you will be on your feet for more than what your knee would normally be able to handle. There are many types of canes, depending on how much support you need. Simple canes offer basic support, while canes with four ground contact points offer added stability for people with decreased strength or balance. The grip on canes vary as well, which is important for people who also have arthritic hands and wrists.

Hiking poles are light, high-tech, functional versions of canes for higher-demand individuals. They can give you support on long hikes on the trails, but can also be used for walks in the city. They are best used as a pair (one in each hand). When used this way, hiking poles will keep your gait even, support both knees simultaneously, and can prevent falls especially when you are traversing rough terrain. Hiking poles are found at sporting goods and outdoor recreation stores.

The most effective way to use a cane is in the hand OPPOSITE to the painful knee. If both knees are painful, you rotate the cane from one hand to the other, or use a pair hiking poles, or use a different assistive device (such as a walker).

When will a walker help me?

A walker provides much more support and stability than a cane. Walkers are most useful when both knees are severely painful, or if there is other pain in the legs or back, or if there are balance issues. Walkers also distribute weight evenly across both arms, for better stability to prevent falls. A walker is good for frail patients, but should be monitored closely because falls can still occur. Even if you usually just use a cane, walkers are good when you need support for a full day of walking and standing.

Some walkers have 2 front wheels and slowly drag forward. Other walkers have 4 wheels with a handbrake for faster walking. Walkers can be prescribed with a built-in seat for sitting down. You can ask your doctor or physical therapist to order a walker from a medical supply store for you.

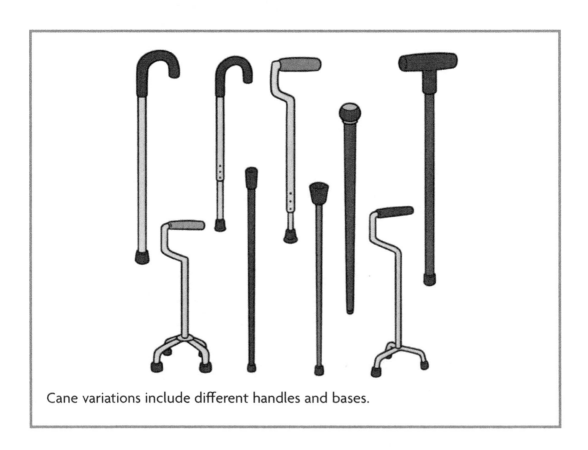

Cane variations include different handles and bases.

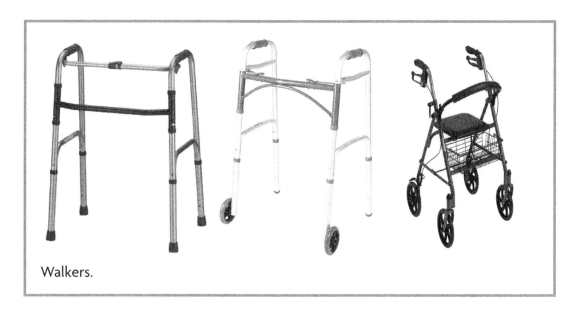

Walkers.

Am I going to end up in a wheelchair?

Your goal in managing your knee OA is to remain as active and independent as possible, preferably on your feet. Although a wheelchair is an available resource for people with knee OA, it is not generally a great option as a long-term intervention. Sitting in a wheelchair will weaken your muscles and decrease your stamina and cardiovascular fitness within just a few days. Once you start depending on a wheelchair, it becomes difficult to return to walking. However, a wheelchair can be very helpful in certain situations for short time periods. For instance, it will help you keep up with your family on a trip to the zoo, and will help you get around the airport quickly and safely. Used strategically, short-term/intermittent usage of a wheelchair can allow you to conserve energy and reduce joint stress to safely get you where you need to be. Some patients have severe OA, or have multiple serious health problems such as dizziness etc. that will not allow them to safely be on their feet. In such cases, wheelchairs may be unavoidable.

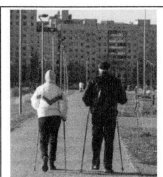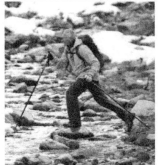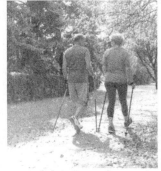

Hiking poles are not just for trekking!! They can help to decrease joint stress, increase endurance, improve balance, and prevent falls.

What if I refuse to use a cane, walker, or wheelchair?

Many people do not want to use a cane or walker because they think that it attracts too much attention, or because it makes them feel old. But assistive devices can be very helpful. For pain flare-ups, assistive devices can take just enough stress off the joints to relieve pain with less intervention. Proactive use of assistive devices can extend the durability of your knees on any given day. And they are not just for "old people". Hiking poles are a great example of a stylish device that can help keep you on the trails longer.

Also, keep in mind that the use of an assistive device may give you the option to participate in activities such as family outings and gatherings rather than staying home. The bottom line is that assistive devices are tools that can be used as needed. You can choose what you use and when you use them. They are totally optional but should be considered if you're having trouble getting around.

MEDICAL TREATMENT 7: "ALTERNATIVE" MEDICINE

Are there any "alternative" treatments for osteoarthritis (OA) that I can discuss with my doctor?

Yes, there are several "alternative" treatments available that do not follow traditional medical theory. The following have been shown in research studies to improve pain and/or function for people with knee OA. Some can be prescribed, and sometimes may be covered by your health insurance. But for the most part the expectation should be that these will be "out of pocket" expenses:

1. **Massage** is manual bodywork designed to soothe and loosen tight, dysfunctional muscles that impair joint movements.
2. **Acupuncture** is an ancient needle-based therapy that triggers pain relief.
3. **Aquatherapy** is water-based physical therapy that is helpful for people who have difficulty with full weightbearing exercise.
4. **Tai chi** consists of a series of slow deliberate movements and postures that can improve balance, strength, and core stability.

You may be wondering about an intervention that isn't listed above. Alternative treatments are always coming and going, but many are unproven, so approach each new trend with caution!

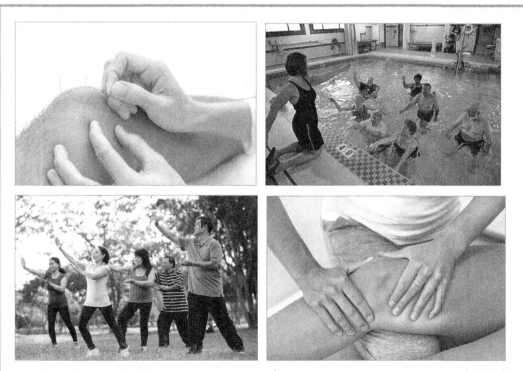

(Clockwise from top left) Acupuncture, aquatherapy, massage treatment, and Tai Chi have proven benefits for people with knee osteoarthritis.

CHAPTER 8
SURGICAL TREATMENTS

Are there surgeries that will treat knee osteoarthritis (OA)?

Yes! There are several surgeries that can treat knee OA. In general, **knee replacement surgery** is the best known, ultimate surgical treatment for knee OA. It is the closest thing to a cure for osteoarthritis. Knee replacement can be considered when the knee is completely worn out ("bone on bone"), with severe pain that has failed conservative treatment. In this procedure, a metal and plastic implant is placed to basically "replace" the entire worn out knee joint.

In certain cases, depending on various factors, other surgeries may be considered:

Osteotomy: This procedure involves cutting bone to realign a knee joint damaged by severe OA. This procedure can allow younger patients a few more years of moderate physical activities while awaiting an eventual total knee replacement.

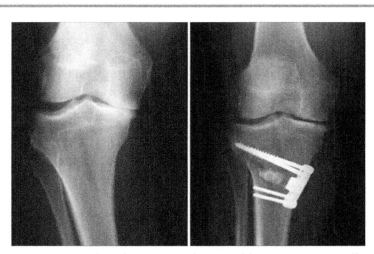

Osteotomy to realign knee joint damaged by joint space collapse.

Partial knee replacement: When painful OA is focused only on one side of the knee joint, it is possible to replace only the arthritic part. People often ask about this option because the implant is smaller and it seems less invasive than total knee replacement. However, this surgery only replaces a part of the joint, and is not helpful if the OA is widespread in the knee. Also, if OA develops elsewhere in the joint after partial replacement, then a full knee replacement may be needed.

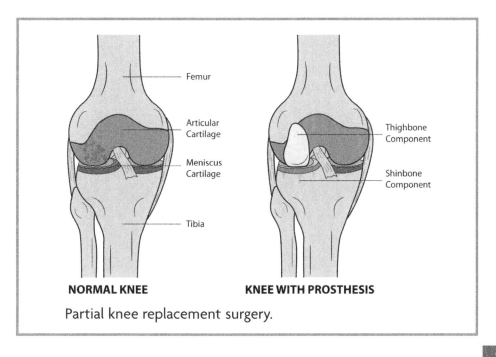

Partial knee replacement surgery.

Patellofemoral (kneecap) joint replacement: In a small percentage of patients, OA is only located where the patella (kneecap) sits on top of the femur (thighbone). The patellofemoral joint can be replaced, providing an option if the rest of the knee is healthy. The affected joint surfaces are replaced with metal and plastic parts. This surgery is less involved than a total knee replacement. However, it only works for the patellofemoral joint, and should not be done if there is also OA elsewhere in the knee.

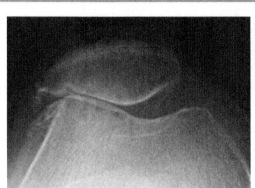 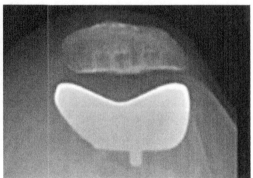

Patellar replacement surgery. There is a plastic component connected to the patella (kneecap) that is not visible on x-ray.

Arthroscopy: Arthroscopy is a minimally invasive surgery that allows access to the knee joint to perform operations without making large incisions. In general, many procedures can be done via arthroscopy. For knee OA, arthroscopy can be utilized to "clean up" damage that has accumulated in the knee. This surgery has become controversial but can be useful in a few specific scenarios.

Cartilage restoration surgery: Although this sounds like a procedure that everyone with OA would want, only certain types of cartilage loss are candidates for an attempt at restoration. Unfortunately, even in ideal conditions, this process is far from perfect, and must be approached with caution.

To summarize, several surgeries are available for knee OA. However, there is no known procedure that can rebuild an arthritic knee to recreate an intact, youthful joint. Surgery requires careful consideration, mostly when conservative measures have failed. Your knee specialist will evaluate your situation and discuss with you the pros/cons and ins/outs of your surgical options. You can get tailor-made advice depending on factors that include your age, symptoms, activity requirements, and the degree of degenerative damage. Surgical outcomes can vary. Even with the best intentions, results cannot be guaranteed and are sometimes unpredictable. Also, surgery cannot be undone if you are dissatisfied with the outcome.

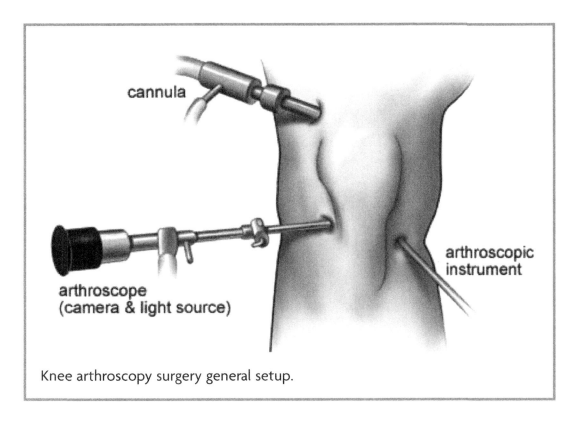

cannula

arthroscopic instrument

arthroscope (camera & light source)

Knee arthroscopy surgery general setup.

What is arthroscopic "cleanup" surgery?

Arthroscopic surgery is a minimally invasive outpatient ("same day") procedure. Small skin incisions are made to create portals that enable a camera and instruments to be inserted into the knee joint. With this setup, a surgeon can perform many different knee operations.

Arthroscopy is an option to treat knee OA but is controversial. Patients frustrated with nagging knee pain from osteoarthritis may want to try arthroscopic surgery for a quick and simple surgical "fix". However, despite what people think, with OA, actual repairs are not usually possible because the cartilage is extensively and irreversibly damaged. The surgeon can only cut away unstable cartilage tears and rough edges, while removing loose pieces. This is called "surgical debridement". Unfortunately, since no rebuilding can be done, the knee will have less cartilage after the procedure.

Medical researchers have found that arthroscopic surgery for osteoarthritis provides mainly temporary relief. In fact, the average benefit of arthroscopy can be as short as a few months, similar to conservative options like a "cortisone" injection. Because arthroscopic debridement causes tissue loss, knee OA can get worse quickly. "Clean-up" arthroscopy for knee OA can lead to knee replacement surgery as soon as one year later. This procedure is most useful when specifically removing unstable cartilage that causes locking or "pinching" in the knee joint that interferes with proper motion and function.

What is total knee replacement surgery?

Total knee replacement surgery (TKR) is a joint resurfacing procedure that is the closest thing to a cure for knee osteoarthritis. First, the arthritic, worn out joint surfaces are cut away. A metal and plastic prosthesis ("bionic joint") is then anchored into the bones to make a new joint. This restores basic function and mechanics to enable pain-free movement.

TKR can be selected when the knee joint is completely worn out from osteoarthritis and conservative (nonsurgical) treatments have failed.

How do I prepare for total knee replacement surgery?

First, medical clearance is needed. Specific conditions that increase risks of complications such as death, disability, infections, and blood clots will need evaluation and treatment before surgery. Once cleared, you can schedule your surgery and start the planning process. You should receive information about how to prepare your home for your recovery. Postoperative home visits for nursing care and physical therapy will be scheduled. Gather a team of family or friends to help you with groceries and simple daily errands when needed. Discuss plans for surgery with your employer so you have a plan for taking time off or modifying your work duties until you are back on your feet.

What is knee replacement surgery like?

The surgery can be done with general anesthesia, where you are "asleep", or with spinal/regional anesthesia where your knee is numb but you are awake. Your surgeon and anesthesiologist will help you decide which option is best for you.

TKR surgery takes about 2 hours. A long vertical incision is made in the front of the leg from above to below the knee. The diseased joint surfaces are removed and the prosthesis is implanted into the bones to make the new artificial joint. This procedure requires cutting and drilling bone. The website for the American Academy of Orthopedic Surgeons (www.aaos.org) has a simple video that gives you a visual understanding of what happens during surgery.

There are many prosthesis variations, made by different manufacturers. You should discuss with your surgeon beforehand which is recommended for you and why. After surgery, most patients will stay in the hospital for up to a few days, but there are now protocols that can safely get patients home as early as the same day of surgery. Once you are home, arrangements should have already been made so that you have the medications, physical therapy, and follow up office visits you will need for a successful, seamless recovery.

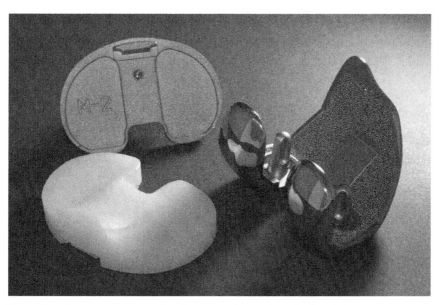

Knee Replacement prosthesis parts (metal and plastic).

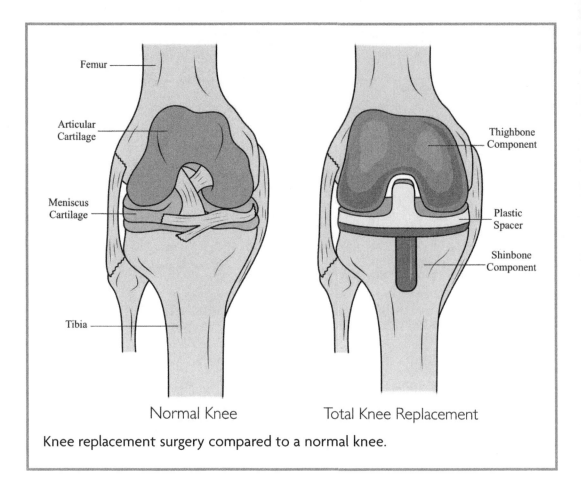

Femur

Articular
Cartilage

Meniscus
Cartilage

Tibia

Thighbone
Component

Plastic
Spacer

Shinbone
Component

Normal Knee   Total Knee Replacement

Knee replacement surgery compared to a normal knee.

What are the risks of knee replacement surgery (TKR)?

TKR is a moderate risk surgery. Your brain, kidneys, heart, lungs, and other organs can get injured because of the general surgical stress on the body. Knee replacement surgery has specific risks of infection, blood clot, bleeding, nerve damage, and persistent pain. The prosthesis is made of metal and plastic thought to be safely hypoallergenic, but the body may reject the implant anyway. Other prosthesis failures can occur, such as loosening or breakdown of the synthetic parts. Anesthesia-related risks can range from mild to annoying to serious. Overall, the risk of complications is about 2 percent, and death from TKR surgery can occur roughly 2 in 1000 times (much less than one percent). The surgical incision can cause minor problems like skin scarring or local nerve damage.

Before your surgery, ask your joint surgeon about how the surgical team will prevent risks and complications. Many hospitals and orthopedic groups have created specific protocols for special safety measures to help ensure patients will have the best outcomes possible.

Is it safe for me to have total knee replacement surgery (TKR)?

There are many medical conditions that can make TKR risky or generally unsafe. You will need medical clearance from your primary care physician and any other specialists who are taking care of ongoing conditions that could affect your surgical risk.

According to orthopedic research, there are 3 specific major health factors that make knee replacement surgery particularly unsafe:
- **uncontrolled diabetes**
- **obesity with BMI greater than 40**
- **tobacco use.**

These must be addressed and resolved before elective TKR surgery is considered.

Is knee replacement surgery painful?

You should expect to have surgical pain from the operation after your procedure, which may last a few days to a few weeks. There can be lingering issues, but fortunately, chronic pain after surgery is uncommon. Ask your surgeon about pain control before you have surgery. Many surgeons now have a special prearranged protocol for postoperative pain management that keep patients comfortable with less narcotic medications. Before you have surgery, ask your surgeon what you should expect for pain control.

What is the recovery time for knee replacement surgery?

Every case varies, but typically it takes several months to recover from knee replacement surgery. Each week along the way there should be improvements. Your surgeon will probably encourage you to get back up on your feet immediately after surgery, but you will be limited to using a walker at first. At

4 to 6 weeks post-surgery you may be walking independently or with a cane. Shortly thereafter you may be able to return to driving, but this will vary per patient. The timeline to return to work will depend on you and your occupation.

Most people should be very functional with activities of daily living around 3 to 6 months after surgery. However, a return to a full schedule that includes sports and hobbies may take longer. It may also take time to become accustomed to the way the new joint feels or moves. For some people, recovery may be very slow, especially if there are surgical complications.

Can I have knee replacement surgery in both knees on the same day?

Maybe. This is a discussion for you and your surgeon. The typical recommendation is to do one knee at a time 3 to 6 months apart, but some patients choose to have both knees operated on the same day. There may be more pain and a longer recovery. Talk to your surgeon about additional risks and considerations.

How successful is knee replacement surgery?

Success can be defined according to two parameters. The technical process of surgically replacing the joint is highly successful when done by an appropriately trained, experienced orthopedic surgeon. The other aspect of success has to do with patient satisfaction with pain relief and return to activities. Knee replacement surgery is most likely to be successful when done in the correct scenario, where you have severe osteoarthritis and have failed nonsurgical treatments. Overall, data shows that roughly 80 percent of people are satisfied with their surgical results. Up to 90 percent of people will experience substantial pain relief. Sources of dissatisfaction include continued pain, limits in function, surgical complications, etc.

How long will the prosthesis last?

Hopefully, a knee replacement will last your lifetime. Current statistics suggest that 80 percent of knee replacements are still functioning 20 years after surgery. However, there is a small percent chance that increases every year after surgery that the prosthesis will fail, requiring some sort of surgical revision.

What age is too old for knee replacement surgery (TKR)?

There is no specific minimum or maximum age for TKR. It is a reasonable option for healthy/low risk patients with severe "bone on bone" OA who have failed conservative care. The current average age of someone having TKR is in the late 60s, but people in their 50s are getting the surgery done more than ever. That said, having TKR surgery at a young age may lead to the need for an eventual revision or replacement of the prosthesis.

Health status, not age, will be the best predictor of whether or not someone should consider TKR. A healthy 90 year old may be medically cleared and have a successful surgery, while a 60 year old may not even be a candidate for surgery because of risky health issues.

Sometimes it is difficult to decide if and when to have knee replacement surgery. It is good to wait, but waiting too long may make the surgery too risky if other health conditions arise in the meantime. Have ongoing conversations with your doctors, and get multiple opinions if needed.

My knees are bad, but I don't want surgery. The rest of my family, however, is insisting I have surgery. What should I do?

Your family may have your best interest in mind. They don't want to see you suffer. They could be right—you may be putting yourself through a lot of pain to avoid surgery. However, ultimately, you are the one that has to undergo a risky procedure, and then live with the results, good or bad. Assuming you are a reasonable surgical candidate, you should only have surgery when you yourself feel you need it. Have open discussions with your doctors, weigh the risks and benefits, and make your own decision.

When should I ask about knee surgery for osteoarthritis(OA)?

You should see an orthopedic surgeon whenever you have questions about what your surgical options are for your knee osteoarthritis. You may go in ready to have surgery, or you may simply want more information. Getting a consultation never means you are automatically signing up for surgery. An in-depth conversation with a specialist can help put your situation into proper perspective. In the meantime, most orthopedic surgeons can offer ongoing medical treatments while you are deciding about surgery.

Keep in mind that not all orthopedic surgeons are the same. A surgeon who is fellowship trained in knee replacement surgery is your go-to for knee replacement, but may not be proficient at doing other procedures for knee OA. You may need to seek consultations from multiple orthopedic surgeons to get the most complete picture of your surgical outlook. Be patient with the process. Write down your questions ahead of time. Take good notes. If your doctor is not patient enough to give you good answers, see someone else. At the same time, be respectful of the surgeon's time and schedule an additional appointment if you have more questions than can be answered in one office visit.

CHAPTER 9
PUTTING A PLAN TOGETHER

Hopefully by now you understand what knee osteoarthritis is and you are becoming familiar with your treatment options. This knowledge empowers you to start creating a plan of action. You can use any or all of the following options:

KNEE OSTEOARTHRITIS TOOLKIT:
Lifestyle changes
Activity modifications
Home treatments
Medications
Injections
Knee braces
Assistive devices
Physical therapy
Alternative treatments
Surgery

That is a pretty big toolkit. How do I know what to choose?

Generally, it's up to you. You can choose to try anything, everything, or nothing on the list. Some people decide to simply deal with their knee pain without any intervention, while others will try everything imaginable. Most people are somewhere in between.

People also vary in how proactive they are in selecting treatment options. Many people take advantage of online resources and word of mouth to gather information, and then pursue treatment accordingly. Meanwhile, others still go the traditional route, letting their doctors decide what to do.

Regardless where you get treatment recommendations, keep track of each option you want to consider. For the treatments that can be done at home on your own, start whenever you are ready. For medical interventions, your primary care physician can help prescribe, administer, or refer accordingly. If you are not sure what to try, get more information. Build a team of healthcare providers that can include an orthopedist, physical therapist, etc. to get the most balanced, comprehensive advice.

How do I know where to begin?

Because you have taken the effort to research your medical condition, you should feel empowered to manage your knee osteoarthritis (OA). Strive to be active in your care. Assemble a team of healthcare providers. Pursue advice and consultations about the treatments that interest you, and keep an open mind when you are presented with new or previously unconsidered options. Then you should be ready to take your first steps.

By now, you probably have an idea where you want to start. If not, then you can begin your treatment journey by using pain as your guide. Most of you should fall into 3 scenarios:

1. *"I don't have much pain; I want a plan to make my knees last as long as possible"*
   This is the most proactive long-term approach: prevent OA-related pain before it becomes a major issue. Your goal here is to "OA-proof" yourself as much as possible. Most of what you do consists of home-based strategies that won't require a doctor's intervention, but your doctor can help support your efforts by monitoring your progress. Decrease your baseline inflammation with a healthy diet. Maintain a safe weight (BMI under 30).

Focus on a clean lifestyle. Consider sensible activity modifications to protect your aging knees even if you are not having pain yet. If you elect to try physical therapy, it should be geared towards a maintenance home program of strength, balance, and stability for better performance, decreased joint stress, and reduced injury risk.

2. *"I regularly get pain, especially whenever I am too active"*
    When your osteoarthritis (OA) flares up from overuse that your knees cannot handle, then painful inflammation will build up. Pain is an important warning signal for OA. The first step is to make adjustments in your activities to reduce ongoing joint stress. Take immediate action. Restrict your activities, including a period of rest, to see if you can get your knees to settle down from being so irritable and easily aggravated. Meanwhile, think about how you will modify your daily routine for the long term to prevent the pain from returning.

    This is also a good time to focus on strategies that will help reduce and prevent inflammation. Get all chronic medical conditions under control to maximize your health. This can improve your body's daily ability to care for itself. Eliminate lifestyle habits that increase inflammation and decrease daily healing. If you are overweight/obese, remember that this is a big contributor for inflammation and chronic OA pain.

    You may need help from your doctor, especially if the knee pain is escalating and difficult to manage on your own. You may need a one-time treatment or ongoing medical management.

3. *" I have pain all the time no matter what I do"*
    If you have severe "wear and tear" in your knees, OA pain may be difficult to control. Plan to see your doctor regularly. Confirm that it is osteoarthritis that is causing your symptoms. Then get ongoing scheduled treatments to get and keep your knee pain under better control. If you can get the pain to resolve, then try to give your knees as much support as possible to better

manage your symptoms. A light physical therapy regimen is helpful for joint support. Assistive devices like a cane, walker, or brace may go a long way in helping you. You may need to schedule injections at regular intervals to keep the pain away.

If you have tried multiple treatments and still aren't getting relief, then you may decide to pursue surgical options.

How do I handle an osteoarthritis(OA) flare-up or a bad day?

This depends on how much pain you are having. If you are having uncontrolled or unmanageable pain, immediately offload your knee and visit your doctor for evaluation. Also remember, if your symptoms seem different than usual, then you should immediately discuss with your doctor to consider other diagnoses because it may not be OA!

For mild flare-ups, you may simply need to slow down or rest for a few days. For more moderate pain and disability, you can use other tools such as assistive devices. Always focus on boosting your diet with healthy foods known to decrease inflammation. In any case, you may want to see your doctor to utilize medical treatments ranging from medications to injections.

As you start to get recover, EASE back into activity at about 25-50% of your usual activity level. Listen closely to what your body is telling you day to day and respect your knee's limitations. Anytime you get sore/achy, it means you will need to make adjustments to slow down further. Your goal should be complete resolution-- do not let your pain linger. If you don't seem to be getting better or if your symptoms keep getting worse, then see your doctor.

NOTE: If you have an accident, fall, or injury that leads to pain, you may have a problem different than your usual OA flare-up. You could have sprained, torn, or broken something. Swelling, escalating pain, an inability to bear weight, or any other issues in this scenario should prompt a visit ASAP to your doctor.

I have seen my doctor, had injections, made modifications, done PT, and nothing really helps for very long—what should I do?

If you feel that you have exhausted your options, then it may be time to start considering surgery. Visit your orthopedic surgeon to review your symptoms, diagnostic imaging, and physical examination to reconfirm your diagnosis of osteoarthritis. You can then discuss your surgical options, including whether or not you are an appropriate candidate for knee replacement.

If you are not interested in or qualified for surgery, or if your doctor tells you it's not time yet, then you could feel like you're in a tough situation. But do not give up! Take another look at the toolkit items. Troubleshoot your diet, lifestyle, and your activities including sports/hobbies/occupation, and home remedies as much as you can. Think about medical interventions you have tried so far such as medications, injections, and physical therapy. Consider items you skipped that maybe worth a second look. Combine and vary treatments until you find a regimen that makes a difference.

If your doctor insists that nothing else can be done, you can't let that be the final word. Take an active approach and regain control of your plan of action. Consider shaking up your medical team with second opinions from other providers to get fresh perspectives and new ideas about your knee pain.

I read the above and I don't feel like any of the above scenarios apply to me. What should I do?

Your personal situation may not fit any of the common patterns that are seen with knee osteoarthritis. Yes, you are an individual and you deserve to be treated like one.

Make an appointment with knee specialists. Discuss your symptoms, goals, and expectations. Get all the required testing done. Make sure you really have osteoarthritis as opposed to some other knee condition.

This book serves as a very basic foundation for your understanding of knee osteoarthritis. This is a starting point for you as an educated healthcare consumer to improve your conversations with your medical providers and make better decisions. During your knee pain journey, you may need to seek more knowledge and information. Talk to experts, read articles, go online, listen to friends and family with arthritis, etc. Your efforts will lead you to become more empowered to be in full control so that you can get the most out of your knees to ensure the quality of life that you deserve.

APPENDIX 1:
SAMPLE HOME EXERCISES

Physical therapy (PT) is very helpful in managing knee osteoarthritis (OA). It is a natural, holistic, medication-free noninvasive treatment. A good PT program for OA will improve function and reduce pain. PT will help preserve your quality of life by keeping you active in your daily activities and favorite sports/hobbies.

It is always best to attend one-on-one PT sessions with a therapist who can evaluate your needs and provide you with exercise sets. Your home program will consist of the following 4 major categories of exercises:

1. Stretching- to improve mobility
2. Strengthening- to increase muscle support to the joint
3. Balance training- to improve single leg mechanics
4. Core stability- to maximize efficiency of leg movement

The sample exercises shown below represent what a home program will look like, from beginner to intermediate/ advanced. These are simply for education and are not intended for diagnosis or treatment of your knee pain. These exercises cannot substitute for seeing and working with a physical therapist. However, if you do not have access to PT, then exercises like these may be better than nothing. Check with your physician to confirm your diagnosis and to make sure it is safe for you to do PT exercises. Whenever you do exercises like these, it is better to be supervised to ensure safety and proper form.

PT SAMPLE EXERCISES

PT EXERCISE CATEGORY 1: STRETCHES

Benefit: prevent stiffness to enable movement.

LEVEL A: BEGINNER

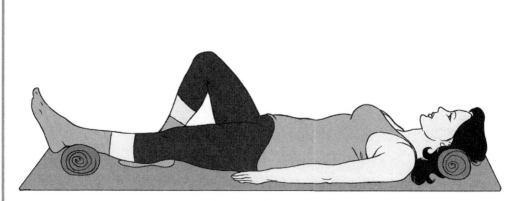

LEG EXTENSION STRETCH

POSITION: Lie on back with rolled up towel under ankle (left leg shown).

EXERCISE: Relax leg to allow knee to naturally extend (straighten) by gravity, hold for 30 seconds.

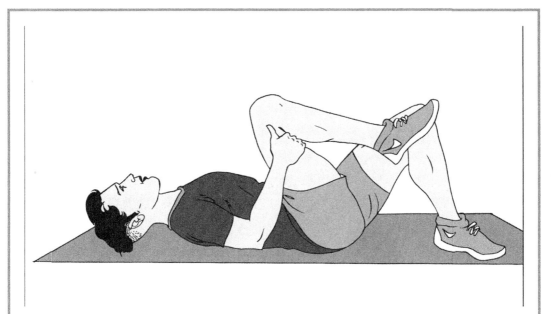

"KNEE TO CHEST" STRETCH

POSITION: Lie on back with both feet flat on ground.

EXERCISE: Raise one leg and pull thigh towards chest as shown, hold for 5 seconds, then repeat 3-5 times each leg.

PT EXERCISE CATEGORY 1:

PT EXERCISE CATEGORY 1: STRETCHES

Benefit: prevent stiffness to enable movement.

LEVEL B: INTERMEDIATE

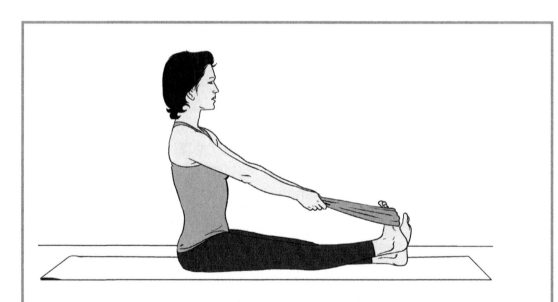

TOWEL STRETCH

POSITION: As shown, holding towel in hands around top of foot.

EXERCISE: Pull towel towards you to feel gentle pull. Hold for 10-15 seconds. Repeat with opposite leg.

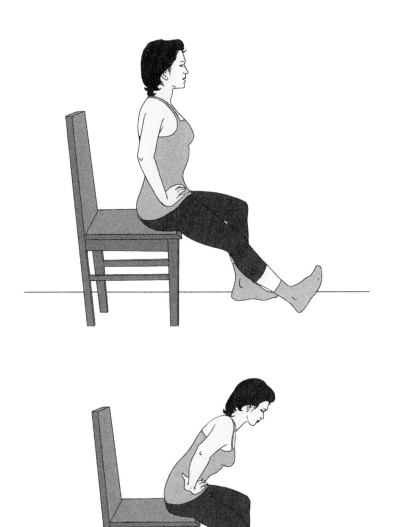

CHAIR HAMSTRING STRETCH

POSITION: Sit at edge of chair with one leg extended (straight).

EXERCISE: Lean forward to feel gentle pull behind thigh in extended leg, and hold for 10-15 seconds. Repeat with opposite leg.

PT EXERCISE CATEGORY 1: STRETCHES

Benefit: prevent stiffness to enable movement.

LEVEL C: ADVANCED

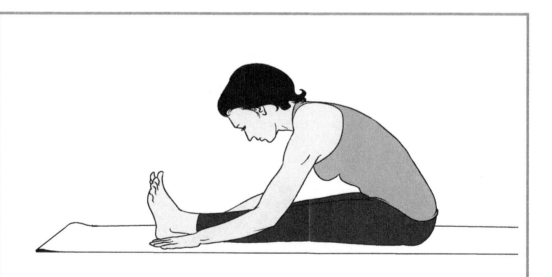

FLOOR HAMSTRING STRETCH

POSITION: Sit on floor, legs straight as shown.

EXERCISE: Lean straight forward to feel gentle pull behind both thighs, hold for 10-15 seconds.

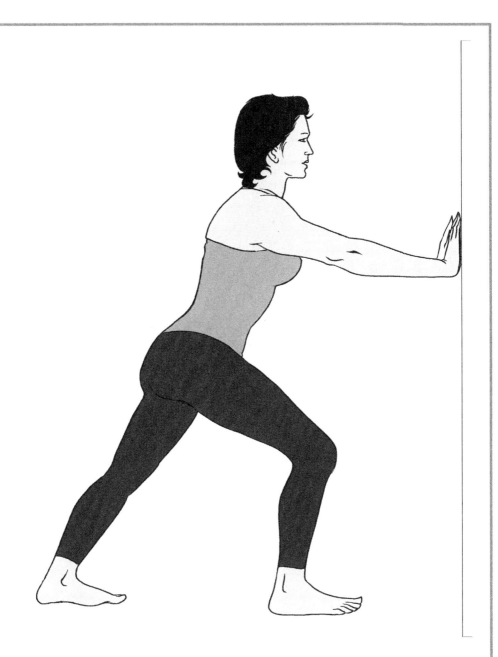

CALF WALL STRETCH

POSITION: Stand facing wall, one foot in front of other, both feet flat on ground.

EXERCISE: Lean forward to feel gentle pull in rear leg, hold for 10-15 seconds. Keep feet flat on ground. Switch legs and repeat.

PT EXERCISE CATEGORY 2: STRENGTH

Benefit: provide muscular support to knee joints.

LEVEL A: BEGINNER

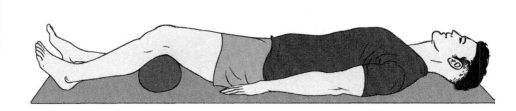

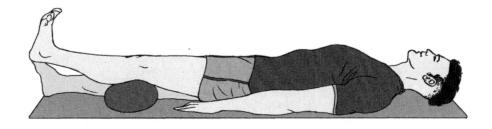

SHORT ARC LEG EXTENSION

POSITION: Lie on back with rolled towel or soft object under knee.

EXERCISE: Lift ankle off ground to straighten knee, hold for 1 second, then return ankle to the ground. Do it again for total of 10 repetitions. Switch legs and repeat.

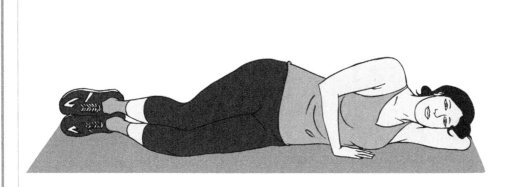

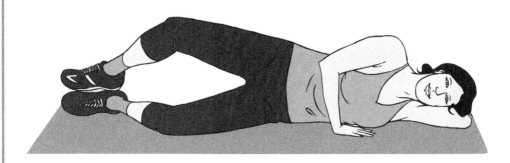

CLAMSHELL EXERCISE

POSITION: Lie on side, knees bent, knees and ankles together.

EXERCISE: Lift knee of top leg while keeping ankles together, and return to starting position. Repeat for total of 5 to 15 repetitions, then switch to lie on opposite side and do it again with the other leg.

PT EXERCISE CATEGORY 2: STRENGTH

Benefit: provide muscular support to knee joints.

LEVEL B: INTERMEDIATE

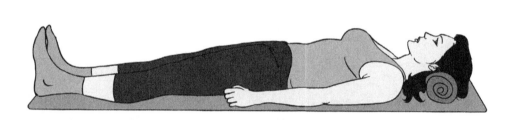

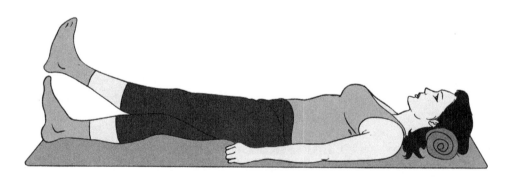

STRAIGHT LEG RAISE EXERCISE

POSITION: Lie on back as shown, legs resting on ground.

EXERCISE: Lift one leg straight up about 6 inches off the ground, then return to starting position. Repeat with other leg. Total 10 repetitions each leg.

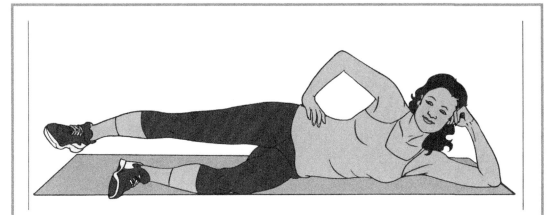

SIDE LYING LEG RAISE EXERCISE

POSITION: Lie on side, bottom leg bent, top leg straight, both feet resting on ground.

EXERCISE: Lift top leg straight up about 6 inches off the ground, then return to starting position. Total 10 repetitions, then turn to opposite side and do the leg lifts with the other leg.

PT EXERCISE CATEGORY 2: STRENGTH

Benefit: provide muscular support to knee joints.

LEVEL C: ADVANCED

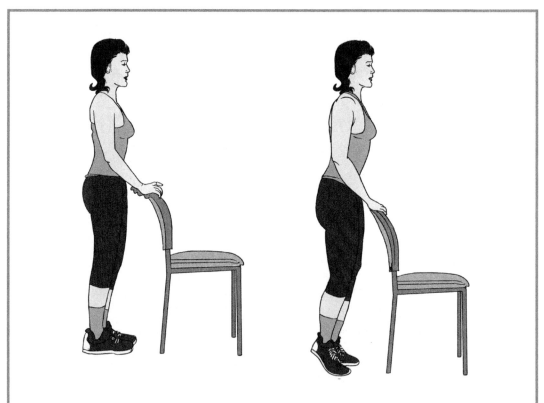

STANDING HEEL RAISE EXERCISE

POSITION: Stand up straight, with feet flat on ground.

EXERCISE: Lift heels 1-2 inches off the ground, then return to starting position. Total 10 repetitions. Hold on to a stationary object for support if needed.

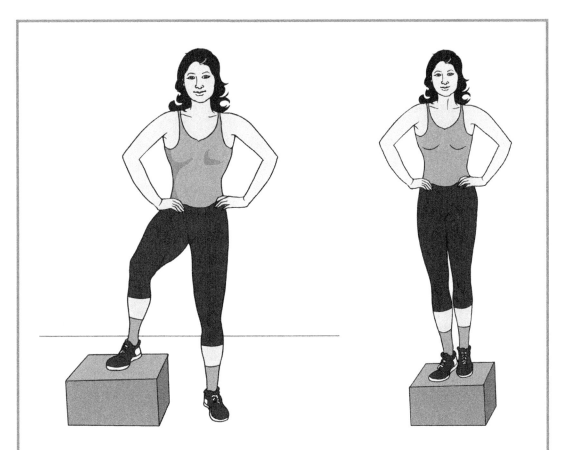

SIDE STEP-UP EXERCISE

POSITION: Stand on step as shown (left).

EXERCISE: Move bottom leg up to step, then return to starting position. Total 10 repetitions, then do exercise with opposite leg on step.

PT EXERCISE CATEGORY 3: BALANCE

Benefit: Improve steadiness, reduce joint stress, prevent falls.

LEVEL A: BEGINNER

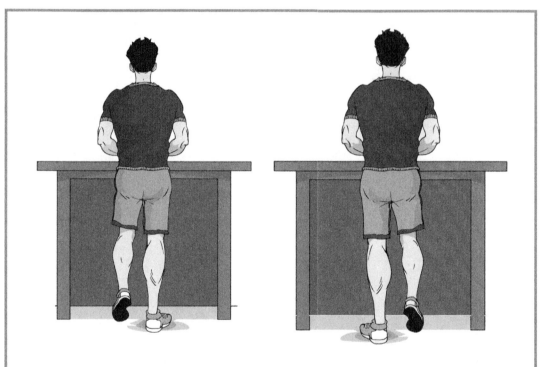

WEIGHT SHIFT EXERCISE

POSITION: Stand in front of table or fixed/stable countertop.

EXERCISE: Shift your weight onto your right leg with your left leg just off the ground for 5 to 10 seconds, holding table/counter for support as needed. Then do the opposite to shift weight onto left leg, again hold for 5-10 seconds. Repeat 3-5 times each leg.

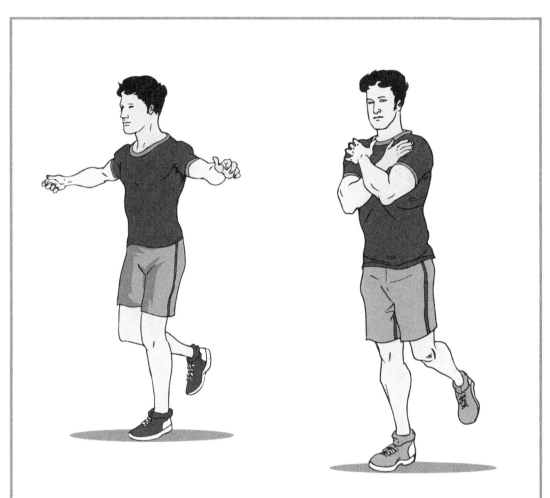

SINGLE LEG BALANCE EXERCISE

POSITION: Stand on a single leg. Intermediate level is with arms extended to help with balance (man on left). Advanced level is with arms crossed (man on right).

EXERCISE: Hold balanced position for as long as possible with goal of 30-60 seconds per leg. **Do exercise near stable object or in doorway where you can catch yourself if you lose your balance during exercise.

PT EXERCISE CATEGORY 3: CORE

Benefit: improve control and efficiency of movement

LEVEL A: BEGINNER

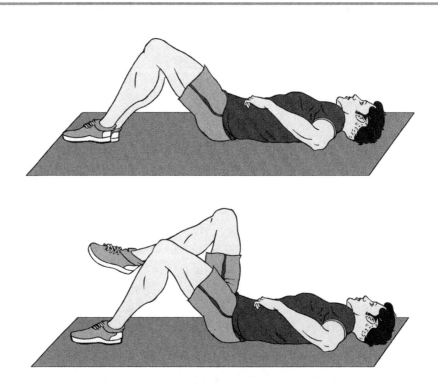

TRUNK EXERCISE 2: LEG RAISE TO BENT KNEE

POSITION: Lie on back on mat, knees bent with feet flat on ground.

EXERCISE: Brace (tighten) trunk and hold. Alternate lifting one leg at a time from straight to bent position a few inches off the ground as shown, and return. Total 10 "marches" each leg, 1-2 sets.

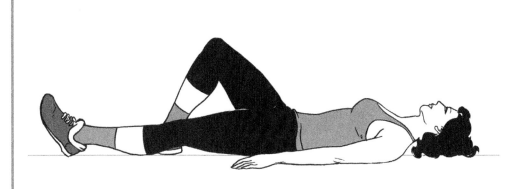

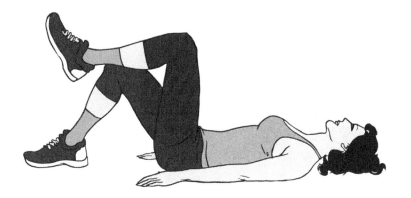

TRUNK EXERCISE 1: SUPINE MARCHES

POSITION: Lie on back on mat, knees bent with feet flat on ground.

EXERCISE: Brace (tighten) trunk and hold. Alternate lifting one foot at a time a few inches off the ground as shown, and return. Total 10 "marches" each leg, 1-2 sets.

BONUS: PERFORMANCE EXERCISES

Benefit: For high-functioning athletes who have osteoarthritis, your therapist can prescribe advanced exercises to better meet your strength/balance/stability needs. Here are some sample exercises.

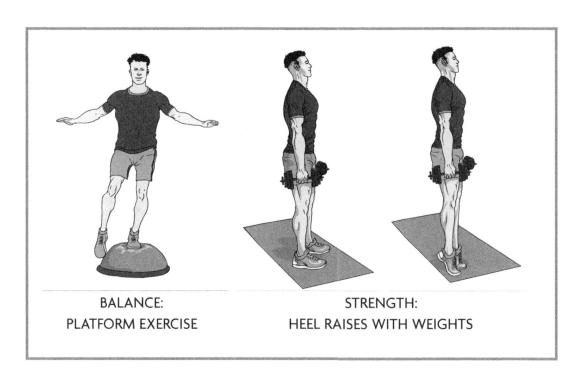

BALANCE:
PLATFORM EXERCISE

STRENGTH:
HEEL RAISES WITH WEIGHTS

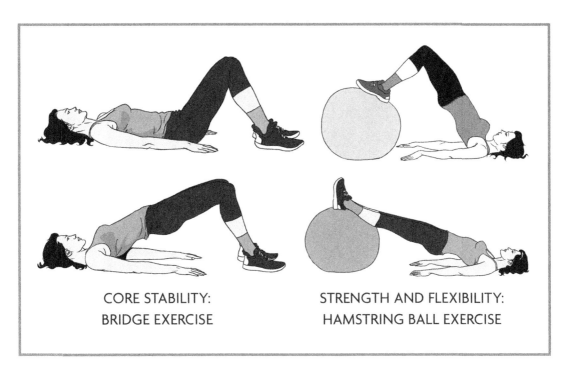

CORE STABILITY:
BRIDGE EXERCISE

STRENGTH AND FLEXIBILITY:
HAMSTRING BALL EXERCISE

APPENDIX 2:
REFERENCES

Adcocks C, Collin P, Buttle DJ. Catechins from green tea (Camellia sinensis) inhibit bovine and human cartilage proteoglycan and type II collagen degradation in vitro. J Nutr. 2002 Mar; 132(3):341-6.

Amin S, Baker K, Niu J, et al. Quadriceps strength and the risk of cartilage loss and symptom progression in knee osteoarthritis. Arthritis and Rheumatism. 2009;60(1):189–198.

Appelboom T, Schuermans J, Verbruggen et al. Symptoms modifying effect of avocado/soybean unsaponifiables (ASU) in knee osteoarthritis. A double blind, prospective, placebo-controlled study. Scand J Rheumatol 2001; 30(4): 242-7.

Bartels EM et al. Aquatic exercise for the treatment of knee and hip osteoarthritis. Cochrane Database Syst Rev 2007; 17 (4): CD005523

Bellamy N et al. Intraarticular corticosteroid for treatment of osteoarthritis of the knee (Review). Cochrane Library 2009, Issue 2.

Bennell K, Hinman R. A review of the clinical evidence for exercise in osteoarthritis in the hip and knee. Jour Sci Med Sport 2011; 14: 4-9.

Berman BM et al. Effectiveness of acupuncture as adjunctive therapy in osteoarthritis of the knee: a randomized, controlled trial. Annals Int Med 2004; 141(12): 901-910.

Bosomworth N. Exercise and knee osteoarthritis: benefit or hazard? Can Fam Phys 2009; 55: 871-878.

Brakke R, Singh J, Sullivan W. Physical Therapy in Persons with Osteoarthritis. P M R 2012; 4: S53-S58.

Bruyere O, Reginster JY. Glucosamine and chondroitin sulfate as therapeutic agents for knee and hip osteoarthritis. Drugs Aging 2007; 24 (7): 573-80.

Brien S et al. Bromelain as a Treatment for Osteoarthritis: a Review of Clinical Studies. Evid Based Complement Alternat Med. 2004 December; 1(3): 251–257.

Brien S, Lewith GT, McGregor G. Devil's claw (Harpagophytum procumbens) as a treatment for osteoarthritis: a review of efficacy and safety. J Altern Complement Med 2006; 12(10): 981-93.

Bruyere O, Pavelka K, Rovati LC, et al. Glucosamine sulfate reduces osteoarthritis progression in postmenopausal women with knee osteoarthritis: evidence from two 3-year studies. Menopause. 2004 Mar-Apr;11(2):138-43.

Buckwalter JA, Lane NE. Does participation in sports cause osteoarthritis? Iowa Orthop J. 1997;17:80–9.

Cadmus L, Patrick MB et l. Community-based aquatic exercise and quality of life in persons with osteoarthritis. Med SCi Sports Exerc 2010; 42 (1): 8-15.

Canter PH, Wider B, Ernst E. The antioxidant vitamins A, C, E and selenium in the treatment of arthritis: a systematic review of randomized clinical trials. Rheumatology (Oxford). 2007 Aug;46(8):1223-33.

Cao L, Zhang XL, Gao YS, Jiang Y. Needle acupuncture for osteoarthritis of the knee: A systematic review and updated meta-analysis. Saudi Med J 2012; 33(5): 526-32.

Childers NF , M Margoles.[3]An Apparent Relation of Nightshades (Solanaceae) to Arthritis Journal of Neurological and Orthopedic Medical Surgery (1993) 12:227-231.

Christensen R., Bartels EM et al. *Effects of weight reduction in obese patients diagnosed with knee osteoarthritis: A systematic review and meta-analysis. Ann Rheum Dis 2007; 66: 433-39.*

Chu, E. *What It Takes To Be Healthy. Dog Ear Publishing, 2007.*

Chyu MC et al. *Complementary and Alternative exercises for management of osteoarthritis. Arthritis [2011, 2011:364319].*

Compher C, Badallino KO. *Obesity and inflammation: Lessons from Bariatric Surgery. J Parenter Enteral Nutr 2008; 32:645-47.*

Cooper C, Snow S, McAlindon TE, Kellingray S, Stuart B, Coggon D, Dieppe PA: *Risk factors for the incidence and progression of radiographic knee osteoarthritis. Arthritis Rheum 2000, 43:995-1000.*

Dandona P, Chaudhuri A, Ghanim H et al. *Anti-inflammatory effects of insulin and the pro-inflammatory effects of glucose. Sem Thoracic Cadrdiovasc Surg 2006; 18 (4): 293-301.*

Deyle et al. *Effectiveness of Manual Physical therapy and exercise in osteoarthritis of the knee. Ann Int Med 2000; 132: 173-81.*

Deyle et al. *Physical therapy treatment effectiveness for osteoarthritis of the knee: a randomized comparison of supervised clinical exercise and manual therapy procedures vs a home exercise program. Phys Ther 2005; 85: 1301-1317.*

DeSilva V, El-Metwally A, Ernst E, et al. *Evidence for the efficacy of complementary and alternative medicines in the management of osteoarthritis: a systematic review. Rheumatology 2011; 50 (5): 911-920.*

Doré et al.: *A longitudinal study of the association between dietary factors, serum lipids, and bone marrow lesions of the knee. Arthritis Research & Therapy 2012 14:R13.*

Esmaillzadeh A, Kimiagar M et al. *Fruit and vegetable intakes, C-reactive protein, and the metabolic syndrome. Am J Clin Nutr December 2006 84: 1489-1497.*

Esposito K and Giugliano D. Whole-grain intake cools down inflammation. Am J Clin Nutr June 2006 83: 1440-1441.

Felson DT, Zhang Y, Hannan MT, Naimark A, Weissman B, Aliabadi P, Levy D: Risk factors for incident radiographic knee osteoarthritis in the elderly: the Framingham Study. Arthritis Rheum 1997, 40:728-733.

Filardo G, Kon E, Buda R, Timoncini A, Di Martino A, Cenacchi A, Fornasari PM, Giannini S, Marcacci M. Platelet-rich plasma intra-articular knee injections for the treatment of degenerative cartilage lesions and osteoarthritis. Knee Surg Sports Traumatol Arthrosc. 2011 Apr; 19(4):528-35. Epub 2010 Aug 26.

Focht BC, Rejeski WJ, Ambrosius WT, Katula JA, Messier SP. Arthritis Rheum. Exercise, self-efficacy, and mobility performance in overweight and obese older adults with knee osteoarthritis. 2005 Oct 15;53(5):659-65.

Gelber AC, Hochberg MC, Mead LA, Wang NY, Wigley FM, Klag MJ: Body mass index in young men and the risk of subsequent knee and hip osteoarthritis. Am J Med 1999, 107:542-548.

Herrlin et al. Arthoscopic or conservative treatment of degenerative medial meniscal tears: a prospective randomised trial. Knee Surg Sports Traumotol Arthrosc 2006; 15(4): 393-401.

Herrlin et al. Is Arthroscopic Surgery beneficial in treating non-traumatic, degenerative medial meniscal tears? A five year follow up. Knee Surg Sports Traumotol Arthrosc 2013; 21(2): 358-64.

Hichberg et al. American College of Rheumatology 2012 Recommendations for the Use of Nonpharmacologic and Pharmacologic Therapies in Osteoarthritis of the Hand, Hip, and Knee. Arthritis Care and Research 2012;64(4): 465-74.

Hochberg MC, Lethbridge-Cejku M, Scott WW Jr, Reichle R, Plato CC, Tobin JD: The association of body weight, body fatness and body fat distribution with osteoarthritis of the knee: data from the Baltimore Longitudinal Study of Aging. J Rheumatol 1995, 22:488-493.

Jordan JM, Luta G, Renner JB, Linder GF, Dragomir A, Hochberg MC, et al. Self-reported functional status in osteoarthritis of the knee in a rural southern community: the role of sociodemographic factors, obesity, and knee pain. Arthritis Care Res. 1996;9(4):273–8.

Jurenka JS.Therapeutic applications of pomegranate (Punica granatum L.): a review. Altern Med Rev. 2008 Jun;13(2):128-44.

Katiyar S, Raman C.Green tea: a new option for the prevention or control of osteoarthritis. Arthritis Res Thery 2011; 13(4): 121.

Katz et al. Surgery vs. Physical Therapy for a meniscal tear and osteoarthritis. NEJM 2013; 368(18): 1675-84.

Kirkeley et al. A Randomized Trial of Arthroscopic Surgery for Osteoarthritis of the Knee. NEJM 2008; 359 (11): 1097-1107.

Koukoulitsa C, Zika C et al. Inhibitory effect of polar oregano extracts on aldolase reductase and soybean lipoxygenase in vitro. Phytotger Res 2006; 20 (7): 605-6.

Kelley DS, Rasooly R, Jacob RA, Kader AA, Mackey BE.. Consumption of Bing sweet cherries lowers circulating concentrations of inflammation markers in healthy men and women. J Nutr. 2006 Apr;136(4):981-6.

Kim, H. J., Barajas, B., Wang, M. and Nel, A. E. (2008) Nrf2 activation by sulforaphane restores the age-related decrease of T(H)1 immunity: role of dendritic cells. J. Allergy Clin. Immunol. 121, 1255-1261.

Kon E, Mandelbaum B, Buda R, Filardo G, Delcogliano M, Timoncini A, Fornasari PM, Giannini S, Marcacci M.Platelet-rich plasma intra-articular injection versus hyaluronic acid viscosupplementation as treatments for cartilage pathology: from early degeneration to osteoarthritis. Arthroscopy. 2011 Nov;27(11):1490-501.

Kujala UM, Kettunen J, Paananen H, Aalto T, Battié MC, Impivaara O, et al. Knee osteoarthritis in former runners, soccer players, weight lifters, and shooters. Arthritis Rheum. 1995;38(4):539–46.

Lansky EP, Newman RA.).Punica granatum (pomegranate) and its potential for prevention and treatment of inflammation and cancer. J Ethnopharmacol. 2007 Jan 19;109(2):177-206.

Last A, Wilson S. Low-Carbohydrate Diets. Am Acad Fam Phys 2006; 73 (11): 1942-48.

Lementowski PW, Zelicoff SB. Obesity and Osteoarthritis. Am J Orthop 2008; 37: 148-151.

Margreth Grotle1,2*, Kare B Hagen1, Bard Natvig1,3, Fredrik A Dahl4 and Tore K Kvien5Obesity and osteoarthritis in knee, hip and/or hand: An epidemiological study in the general population with 10 years follow-up. BMC Musculoskeletal Disorders 2008, 9:132.

Liu S., Manson J.E., Buring J.E., et al: Relation between a diet with a high glycemic load and plasma concentrations of high-sensitivity C-reactive protein in middle-aged women. Am J Clin Nutr 2002; 75:492-498.

Lopez HL. Nutritional interventions to prevent and treat osteoarthritis. Part II focus on micronutrients and supportive nutraceuticals. PMR 2012 May; 4 (5 suppl):s155-68.

Lopez HL. Nutritional interventions to prevent and treat osteoarthritis. Part I: focus on fatty acids and macronutrients. PM R. 2012 May;4(5 Suppl):S145-54.

Lopez-Garcia E, Schulze MB. Major dietary patterns are related to plasma concentrations of markers of inflammation and endothelial dysfunction.Am J Clin Nutr October 2004 80: 1029-1035.

Lutsey PL, Jacobs DR Jr, Kori S, Mayer-Davis E, Shea S, Steffen LM, Szklo M, Tracy R. Whole grain intake and its cross-sectional association with obesity, insulin resistance, inflammation, diabetes and subclinical CVD: The MESA Study. Br J Nutr. 2007 Aug;98(2):397-405.

Masters RC, Liese AD, Haffner SM, Wagenknecht LE, Hanley AJ. Whole and refined grain intakes are related to inflammatory protein concentrations in human plasma.J Nutr. 2010 Mar;140(3):587-94. Epub 2010 Jan.

Mavrommatis CI, Argyra E, Vadalouka A, Vasilakos DG. *Acupuncture as an adjunctive therapy to pharmacological treatment in patients with chronic pain due to osteoarthritis of the knee: a 3-armed randomized, placebo-controlled trial. Pain 2012 153(8): 1720-6.*

McAlindon TE, Wilson PW, Aliabadi P, Weissman B, Felson DT. *Level of physical activity and the risk of radiographic and symptomatic knee osteoarthritis in the elderly: the Framingham Study. Am J Med. 1999;106(2):151–7.*

Messier SP. *Obesity and osteoarthritis: Disease genesis and nonpharmacologic weight management, Rheum Dis Clin North Am 2008; 34: 713-729.*

Messier SP, Loeser RF, Miller GD, Morgan TM, Rejeski WJ, Sevick MA, Ettinger WH Jr, Pahor M, Williamson JD *Exercise and dietary weight loss in overweight and obese older adults with knee osteoarthritis: the Arthritis, Diet, and Activity Promotion Trial. Arthritis Rheum. 2004 May;50(5):1501-10.*

Michel BA, Stucki G, Frey D, et al. *Chondroitins 4 and 6 sulfate in osteoarthritis of the knee: a randomized, controlled trial. Arthritis Rheum. 2005 Mar;52(3):779-86.*

Morris A et al. *Sleep Quality and Duration are Associated with Higher Levels of Inflammatory Biomarkers: the META-Health Study. Circulation ; 122: A17806.*

Moseley et al. *A Controlled Trial of Arthroscopic Surgery for Osteoarthritis of the Knee. NEJM 2002; 347: 81-8.*

Nanri A, Yoshida D, et al. *Dietary patterns and C-reactive protein in Japanese men and women. Am J Clin Nutr May 2008 87: 1488-1496*

Neogi T, Booth SL, Zhang YQ, et al. *Low vitamin K status is associated with osteoarthritis in the hand and knee. Arthritis Rheum 2006;54:1255–61.*

Otterness IG, Eskra JD, Bliven ML, Shay AK, Pelletier JP, Milici AJ. *Exercise protects against articular cartilage degeneration in the hamster. Arthritis and Rheumatism. 1998;41(11):2068–2076.*

Paans N, van den Akker-Scheek I et al. *Effect of Exercise and Weight Loss in Patients with Hip Osteoarthritis Who are Overweight or Obese: A Prospective Cohort Study.* Phys Ther Sept 2012 epub.

Pavelka K, Gatterova J, Olejarova M, et al. *Glucosamine sulfate use and delay of progression of knee osteoarthritis: a 3-year, randomized, placebo-controlled, double-blind study.* Arch Intern Med. 2002 Oct;162(18):2113-23.

Pelletier JP, Martel-Pelletier J, Abramson SB.*Osteoarthritis, an inflammatory disease: potential implication for the selection of new therapeutic targets.* Arthritis Rheum. 2001 Jun;44(6):1237-47.

Perlman AI, Williams AL et al. *Massage therapy for osteoarthritis of the knee: a randomized controlled trial.* Arch Int Med 2006; 166(22): 2533-38.

Perlman AI et al. *Massage therapy for osteoarthritis of the knee: a randomized dose-finding trial.* PLoS One 2012 7(2): e30248.

Piercarlo Sarzi-Puttini, Marco A. Cimmino, Raffaele Scarpa, Roberto Caporali, Fabio Parazzini, Augusto Zaninelli, Fabiola Atzeni, Bianca Canesi*Osteoarthritis: An Overview of the Disease and Its Treatment Strategies* Seminars in Arthritis and Rheumatism Volume 35, Issue 1, Supplement 1 , Pages 1-10, August 2005.

Qi L, van Dam RM, Liu S, Franz M, Mantzoros C, Hu FB. *Whole-grain, bran, and cereal fiber intakes and markers of systemic inflammation in diabetic women.* Diabetes Care. 2006 Feb; 29(2):207-11.

Rabago D et al. *Hypertonic dextrose injections (prolotherapy) for knee osteoarthritis: results of a single-arm uncontrolled study with 1-year follow-up.* J Altern Complement Med 2012; 18(4): 408-14.

Reeves K, Hassanein K. *Randomized Prospective Double-Blind Placebo-Controlled Study of Dextrose Prolotherapy for Knee OAteoarthritis with or without ACL Laxity.* Alt Ther 2000 6(2): 68-80.

Reginster JY, Deroisy R, Rovati LC, et al. *Long-term effects of glucosamine sulphate on osteoarthritis progression: a randomised, placebo-controlled clinical trial.* Lancet. 2001 Jan;357(9252):251-6.

Reginster JY, Kahan A, Vignon E. A two-year prospective, randomized, double-blind, controlled study assessing the ef- fect of chondroitin 4&6 sulfate (CS) on the structural progres- sion of knee osteoarthritis: STOPP (STudy on osteoarthritis progression prevention). American College of Rheumatology Scientific Meeting 2006;(online abstract).

Reijman M, Pols HA, Bergink AP, Hazes JM, Belo JN, Lievense AM, Bierma-Zeinstra SM: Body mass index associated with onset and progression of osteoarthritis of the knee but not of the hip. The Rotterdam Study. Ann Rheum Dis 2007, 66:158-62.

Roos H, Lindberg H, Gärdsell P, Lohmander LS, Wingstrand H. The prevalence of gonarthrosis and its relation to meniscectomy in former soccer players. Am J Sports Med. 1994;22(2):219–22.

Rosenbaum C et al. Antioxidants and Antiinflammatory Dietary Supplements for Osteoarthritis and Rheumatoid Arthritis. Alt Ther 2010; 16(2): 32-40.

Salas-Salvadó J, Casas-Agustench P, Murphy MM, López-Uriarte P, Bulló M. The effect of nuts on inflammation. Asia Pac J Clin Nutr. 2008;17 Suppl 1:333-6.

Sampson S, Reed M, Silvers H, Meng M, Mandelbaum B. Injection of platelet-rich plasma in patients with primary and secondary knee osteoarthritis: a pilot study. Am J Phys Med Rehabil. 2010 Dec;89(12):961-9.

Schulze MB, Hoffmann K et al. Dietary pattern, inflammation, and incidence of type 2 diabetes in women. Am J Clin Nutr September 2005 82: 675-684

Seki T, Hasegawa Y, Yamaguchi J, Kanoh T, Ishiguro N, Tsuboi M, Ito Y, Hamajima N, Suzuki K. Association of serum carotenoids, retinol, and tocopherols with radiographic knee osteoarthritis: possible risk factors in rural Japanese inhabitants. .J Orthop Sci. 2010 Jul;15(4):477-84.

Selfe TK, Taylor AG. Acupuncture and osteoarthritis of the knee: a review of randomized controlled trials. Family and Community Health 2008; 31(3_: 247-54.

Sharif M, Shepstone L, Elson CJ et al. Increased C-Reactive Protein may reflect events that precede radiographic progression in OA of the knee. Ann Rheum Dis 2000; 59: 71-74.

Sharma L, Pai YC. Impaired proprioception and osteoarthritis. Curr Opin Rheumatol. 1997;9(3):253–8.

Shen CL, Smith BJ, et al. Dietary Polyphenols and mechanisms of osteoarthritis. J Nutr Biochem 2012 Nov; 23(11): 1367-77.

Shrager MA, Metter EJ et al. Sarcopenic obesity and inflammation in the InCHianti Study. J Appl Physiol 2007; 102: 919-925.

Sihoven et al. Arthroscopic Partial Meniscectomy vs. Sham Surgery for a Degenerative Meniscal Tear. NEJM 2013; 369: 2515.

Sihvonen R et al. Mechanical Symptoms and Arthoscopic Partial Meniscectomy in Patients with Degenerative Meniscus Tear: A Secondary Analysis of a Randomized Trial. Ann Int Med 164(7): 449-55.

Spector TD, Hart DJ, Doyle DV: Incidence and progression of osteoarthritis in women with unilateral knee disease in the general population: the effect of obesity. Ann Rheum Dis 1994, 53:565-568.

Spector TD, Hart DJ et al. Low-level increases in serum C-reactive protein are present in early osteoarthritis of the knee and predict progressive disease. Arthritis Rheum 1997; 40: 723-27.

Spector TD, Hart DJ, Nandra D, Doyle DV, Mackillop N, Gallimore JR, Pepys MB. Low-level increases in serum C-reactive protein are present in early osteoarthritis of the knee and predict progressive disease. Arthritis Rheum. 1997 Apr;40(4):723-7.

Stensrud et al. A 12-week exercise therapy program in middle-aged patients with degenerative meniscus tears: a case series with 1-year follow up. JOSPT 2012; 42(11): 911-31.

Sturmer T, Brenner H, Koenig W, Gunther KP. *Severity and extent of osteoarthritis and low grade systemic inflammation as assessed by high sensitivity C reactive protein. Ann Rheum Dis. 2004, 63: 200-205.*

Sutton AJ, Muir KR, Mockett S, Fentem P. *A case-control study to investigate the relation between low and moderate levels of physical activity and osteoarthritis of the knee using data collected as part of the Allied Dunbar National Fitness Survey. Ann Rheum Dis. 2001;60(8):756–64.*

Tangvoranuntakul P, Gagneux P, Diaz S. et al. *Human uptake and incorporation of an immunogenic nonhuman dietary sialic acid. PNAS 2003 100 (21) 12045-12050.*

Uebelhart D, Malaise M, Marcolongo R, et al. *Intermittent treatment of knee osteoarthritis with oral chondroitin sulfate: a one-year, randomized, double-blind, multicenter study versus placebo. Osteoarthritis Cartilage. 2004 Apr;12(4):269-76.*

Valderrabano V, Steiger C. *Treatment and Prevention of Osteoarthritis through Exercise and Sport. Jour Aging Research 2011.*

Valtueña S et al. *Food selection based on total antioxidant capacity can modify antioxidant intake, systemic inflammation, and liver function without altering markers of oxidative stress. Am J Clin Nutr May 2008 87: 1290-1297.*

van Baar et al. *Effectiveness of exercise therapy in patients with osteoarthritis of the hip or knee. Arthritis and Rheumatism 1999; 42(7): 1361-9.*

Vincent HK, Heywood et al. *Obesity and Weight Loss in the Treatment and Prevention of Osteoarthritis. AAPMR2012, 4:S59-S67.*

Wang S, Olson-Kellog B, et al. *Physical Therapy Interventions for Knee Pain Secondary to Osteoarthritis: A Systematic Review. Ann Int Med 2012; 157 (9): 632-45.*

Wang Y, Wluka AE, Hodge AM, English DR, Giles GG, O'Sullivan R, Cicuttini FM: *Effect of fatty acids on bone marrow lesions and knee cartilage in healthy, middle-aged subjects without clinical knee osteoarthritis. Osteoarthritis Cartilage 2008, 16:579-83.*

Wang Y, Hodge AM, Wluka AE, English DR, Giles GG, O'Sullivan R, Forbes A, Cicuttini FM.Effect of antioxidants on knee cartilage and bone in healthy, middle-aged subjects: a cross-sectional study. . Arthritis Res Ther. 2007;9(4):R66.

Woolf AD, Breedveld FC, Kvien TK: Controlling the obesity epidemic is important for maintaining musculoskeletal health. Ann Rheum Dis 2006, 65:1401-1404.

Yang CS, Landau JM. Effects of tea consumption on nutrition and health. J Nutr. 2000 Oct;130(10):2409-12.

Yim et al. A Comparative Study of Meniscectomy and Nonoperative Treatment for Degenerative Horizontal Tears of the Medial Meniscus. AJSM 2013; 41(7): 1565-70.

Printed in Great Britain
by Amazon

25585399R00077